# Joey Somebody

The Life and Times of a Recovering Douchebag

# Joey Somebody

The Life and Times of a Recovering Douchebag

## Joey Dumont and Paul Dumont

True Thirty, LLC

San Francisco, CA

True Thirty, LLC
San Francisco, CA

www.joeydumont.com

Publisher's Note: This book is memoir. It reflects the author's present recollections of experiences over time. Some names and characteristics have been changed, some events have been compressed, and some dialogue has been recreated.

Design © 2021 Justin Wambolt-Reynolds

First Edition

ISBN 978-1-7368784-2-2 (hardcover)
ISBN 978-1-7368784-1-5 (paperback)
ISBN 978-1-7368784-0-8 (ebook)

To my little boys, Kingston and Kannon, so that you will understand that even your heroes are vulnerable.

— Daddy

In loving memory of Steven James Dumont
(January 1, 1973 – April 10, 2007)

— Paul

# Acknowledgement

_____

To my wife, Debbie, who defines what it means to be the better half. And without whom, there would be no Joey Somebody–only an aging douchebag. She was the motivation for me to become a better man. She's the greatest Mommy in the world. A cherished daughter and sister. A best friend to many. An accomplished executive. And the kindest human being I know.

You are reading this book because of her. And me. And Paul. But mostly her.

# Contents

# Joey Somebody

The Life and Times of a Recovering Douchebag

# Prologue

---

## "I am a Douchebag"
### (2014)

I'm running late. Five-hundred-and-eighteen snorting horses nudge my two-ton sports sedan down the busy Ninth Street off-ramp into San Francisco, twin car seats framing the back row, Cheddar Bunnies and Cheerios smashed into my quilted leather upholstery. My liquid dashboard announces two incoming calls: the boys' preschool headmistress, whose impending tardiness reminder would include admonishments in Mandarin; and my wife, Debbie, whose words carried by cell towers from an Orlando hotel room would arrive solely in English. *Sorry, babe. On my way. Completely my fault. Yes, the boys come first. Yes, I am driving carefully. Won't happen again. Have fun in Florida. Love you, too.*

By the time I respond to both calls, I'm roaring down Ninth toward Russian Hill. I bypass Van Ness and cut into the Tenderloin district, San Francisco's proverbial grease trap, infamous for its brackish sea-level buildings with cracked windows and spray paint, padlocked Porta Potties, weak streams of piss flowing over shit-smeared sidewalks, ironic shopping carts, wheeled walkers, Rascal scooters, clicking canes, cigarettes, and addicts in overcoats shuffling in circles attempting to eat their own mouths. Tourists avoid these streets.

I accelerate up the potholed pavement of Larkin Street while avoiding the stoned jaywalkers popping out like shooting gallery targets. But as I cut around a braking Uber driver, intending to accelerate through the intersection, the stale yellow light flips to red, causing me to stomp on the brake pedal like Fred Flintstone. My low-pro tires shriek and spit stones at people near the crosswalk, the stink of burnt carbon and middle-aged arrogance now commingling and ascending with the scuffed dust of the street.

"WHO THE FUCK DO YOU THINK YOU ARE?" I look over my left shoulder to see three men, each twice my mass and masculinity, now approaching my car with the slow confidence of magma: large-knuckled meat hands, tattooed fingers with thick metal rings, spotless Timberland boots, and the smell of low-grade weed and alcohol trailing their exclamation like thunder stumbles after lightning. I slowly lean out my open driver's side window, tilt my head upward to meet their riled eyes, and say, "I . . . AM A DOUCHEBAG, AND I'M SORRY." Which immediately causes the leader to laugh out loud while stomping his big boot twice. I burst out laughing too—with relief— because two seconds prior, I was expecting to be ripped out of my intact seat belt, spiked to the pavement, and pummeled like a Russian protester. Instead, this very large young man extends his open palm and says, "*That* was awesome, dude . . . *You* are awesome!"

In male speak, a douchebag is an overreaching tool—two insults in a single word. A tool is a low-functioning person who by definition is unaware of his limitations. The douchebag, on the other hand, is a tool laboring under a transparent facade of arrogance and grandiosity, like a spoiled media executive who frightens his neighbors by driving like an asshole. My wife hates the word douchebag. My mother would call it dirty. My therapist told me it was a breakthrough.

# Chapter 1

---

## Stevie
### (April 2007)

My baby brother's casket floated like an apparition, the altar enlarging as we moved slowly down the aisle of St. Francis Catholic Church, where decades earlier my brothers and I had devoted our spiritual energies each Sunday to provoking burst of laughter from one another—and in the best-case scenario, a fart—reaping the pinched-face anger of our mortified mother and her sermonized threats of eternal damnation on the drive home. Mom, balancing on her little tiny feet, shuffled ahead of me, flanked by her second poorly chosen husband, intermittent sobs shuddering her bent frame nearer to collapse. Next to me, my remaining brother, Paul, was a statue of tearless rage. Seated alone in the front pew, with his congested heart and shriveled beans for kidneys, medicine ball belly and sausage-link extremities, my father honored his youngest son's memory by furtively filling his adult diaper with last night's bereavement dinner of a whole buttered lobster, puck-sized crab cakes, and a guzzled bottle of white zinfandel. Hundreds of friends and relatives stood still and straight like the blades of frozen grass emerging from the thawing ground of April in Minnesota.

I answered my cell phone during the procession to field a call from my business partners as they raced down Highway 52 updating me on their imminent arrival after they jumped on a last-minute redeye to Minneapolis. I sat in the first pew. I was told that I had delivered the eulogy. The only thing I remember about the mass is that I had too much time to think. Later, I observed Paul watching Stevie's casket being loaded into the hearse, his feet moving slightly as if he were about to chase after it. Consoling souls crammed into the church basement. Mom was stood up in a scrum of sympathy. Old ladies shepherded cold cuts and hot dishes between a bright kitchen and brimming buffet table while neighbors and relatives I had trouble recognizing attempted to hug away my pain. I noticed the attendance of Stevie's first wife, but not his second. Childhood friends in their mid-thirties. A few of Stevie's fellow outpatients from surrounding treatment centers. An afternoon of slow-motion consolations. No happily ever after.

Between his high school graduation in June 1991, and his death on April 10, 2007, Steven James Dumont relocated dozens of times across four states, embarrassed a half dozen rehabilitation centers, failed panels of sobriety tests, incurred at least four DUIs, celebrated the holidays in county jails and detention centers, and secured and lost over forty-five low-paying jobs. Any income he earned was consumed in rapacious gulps by lost security deposits, moving expenses and reactivation fees, and retail alcohol and black-market drug prices—all logical consequences of ingesting copious amounts of vodka, other misappropriated spirits, and low-quality marijuana since elementary school. Stevie complemented his alcohol consumption by introducing a panoply of more dangerous narcotics into his coping regimen: bindles of methamphetamine and heroin, orange bottles of opioids and other "prescription" medications with childhood safety caps, and inhalants, or "huffing."

Stevie's marriages were catastrophes. Stevie's first wife, Ashley, was a beautiful woman twenty-four months out of high school with a methamphetamine habit that controlled the remainder of her life. Fortunately, this marriage—riddled with stimulant-addled sexual dysfunction and acts of domestic violence, anxious incompetence, chronic unemployment, congested ashtrays and empty refrigerators, and finally a well-deserved eviction notice—lasted only eleven months and did not produce any children. Stevie's second wife, Sharon, was close to her family and her religion, a member of the military, and a recent college graduate whose ridiculous decision to marry an unemployed drug addict implied a previously unplumbed wellspring of willful ignorance and unbridled arrogance. While my family, during the drive to the wedding in Iowa, devoted ample conversation to the marriage's impending demise, it was Sharon's father who later best encapsulated the moment, sitting in the front pew of the tiny rent-a-church, bent over in crash position clutching his head with both hands as if his daughter was marrying her own brother. This marriage crashed and burned in less than two years.

In hindsight, Stevie was doomed and broken and he couldn't be put back together, making our desperate family intervention, conducted less than three hundred days before his death, no more than an absurdity, like throwing a towel to a drowning man. Unable to appreciate the contributory roles of imperfect actors, Stevie blamed himself for his addiction and arrested development, directing his frustration and resultant aggression inward as though he believed he could fill the hole in his soul with enough suffering to lift him back to solid ground. Stevie spent the final decade of his life cycling through rehabilitation programs, detention facilities, dark apartments, and Mom's basement bedroom. Like a rock star touring facilities across Minnesota, he flowed among the broken and forgotten, held aloft by like-kind addicts diverted to the gutters and sewers. As if he believed that was where he belonged.

Unable to name his pain, Stevie died quietly.

# Chapter 2

## Silver Spoon
### (June 1974–February 1982)

Saturday afternoon. I'm seven years old, post-breakfast, splayed face down, hanging off the edge of my unmade bed in a fresh T-shirt and cut-off shorts. Bare feet, languid arm drifting toys in the direction of a babbling toddler Stevie with sun-browned skin and a shock of curly dark hair in a pressed blue sunsuit and clean cloth diaper. My bespectacled, same-sized brother Paul—less than a year older than me—is propped on his side lost in a comic book, one skinny leg tucked under a sheet. We are supposed to be cleaning our room. Mom's staccato steps reverberate in bursts as she attacks all of the housework at the same time, pinballing between floors and rooms of our ranch-style starter home, one of the first built in a new Rochester, MN hilltop neighborhood populated by young families led by doctors, engineers, and other professionals. Northern Heights. "The Hill." One hundred yards from our elementary school and a mile from the Mayo Clinic. Acres of newly planted trees.

An engine's nasal rage interrupts. I smile at my brothers: "Let's go, guys!" Scoop up Stevie. Seconds later we smack past the front screen door, navigate the stairs, cross the black-tarred driveway, and sprint around the garage into the backyard to skip behind Dad in the wake of the lawnmower, singing *Follow the Yellow Brick Road*, the crew-cut grass massaging cool between warm bare toes. Afterward, we play baseball with a white plastic ball and *Fat Albert* bat. Dig holes in the sand-filled tractor tire. Run through sparkling sprinklers across fenceless backyards. Climb on pendulum swing sets. Share hot dogs and burgers with bugs at our splintered picnic table. Neighborhood sunset hide-and-seek. "Olly olly oxen free!" Baths. Bedtime stories. Night-lights. Summer days with our friends at the bottom of the driveway digging dirt roads into the soft curbside for our Hot Wheels and Matchbox cars. Chalk cities on driveways and the basement floor. Legions of "paper people," self-drawn cutout DC and Marvel action figures colored in crayon that we sent on countless adventures. Board games. Play money. Soda pop, darts, and cap guns. Cereal box nutrition information contests involving Iron, Riboflavin, and Zinc, with Total and King Vitamin acting as ringers. Fighting over the blue bowl.

My earlier memories depicted a smaller family, before Stevie was born, lost recollections chronicled and reinforced through Mom's regular contributions to the big brown family album. The earliest photos captured four Dumonts in the act of life and every possible relational permutation: me, Mom, Dad, and Paul standing in front of Grandpa's VW microbus outside Great Aunt Mary's home in South Dakota. Or with Uncle Pat's family and our grandparents in Prior Lake. Or together at Yosemite National Park. There was Mom and Dad's wedding in 1962 at the big church in Mom's hometown of Easton, Minnesota. Mom holding Paul. Dad holding me on a motorcycle. Many of me and Paul in clean outfits and pajamas. Me and Mom. Paul and Dad. More of me and Paul. Lots of blue-sky backgrounds. A nice Minnesota family.

But the album told another story. Halfway through, photos of an infant Stevie appeared: Stevie just home from the hospital wrapped in Mom's arms; Stevie posing in his crib with his blond Baby Beans doll; scores of shots of Stevie, Paul, and me, Stevie always in the middle. Big smiles. Blue skies. Yet no photos of the five of us. I have yet to find a snapshot showcasing Mom, Dad, Paul, me, and Stevie in the archetypal proud family portrait poses I saw mounted in living rooms or magnetized to my friends' refrigerators. No thousand-word pictures of Dad and Stevie together. No photos of just Mom and Dad looking happily at the camera. Something didn't look right.

That summer, after we were expected to fall asleep, even Stevie could detect Mom and Dad's increasingly frequent after-dark muffled clashes of raw emotion and exigency, quickened and ominous dramas—Dad's long, calm cadences interspersed with Mom's sharp replies. Tones of impending sorrow. Bad dreams. In August, Dad made a mysterious ten-day trip. He returned with tanned skin, an unnecessary haircut, hip new clothes, designer sunglasses, and a shiny pastel-green American Express card. Bouncing with excitement, he gushed about the bosomy beauty of California's Bay Area. He brought us eclectic presents, including "I Heart San Francisco" T-shirts, miniature cable cars, and a vinyl forty-five of Harry Chapin's "Cats in The Cradle." Irony marked the end of my childhood.

Dad bugged out a few weeks later, speeding away in his company car with only a few suitcases, leaving behind a young wife and three sons, his parents and siblings, his colleagues and neighbors, and his church. He signed papers assigning ownership of his pristine single-family residence to Mom, provided she assumed the mortgage and remaining seventeen years of parenting duties. He began contributing $16.67 per day. In two monthly installments. The phone explained to us in Dad's voice that he had accepted a job transfer for the good of the family and that we would all follow him to the West Coast that following summer. Be put back together. This explanation made sense. Neighborhood families with brilliant fathers who worked for IBM were regularly transferred across the country. Relocating was a sign of success and status. Maybe Dad was brilliant. We told our friends and teachers we were moving to the Golden State. Hardly a word from Mom.

We flew out to California in June of 1975; it was everyone's first ride on a plane. Mom looked sick and terrified, but my brothers and I were tanked with excitement throughout the four-hour flight. At the gate, Mom and Dad kind of hugged each other. Dad was glad to see us. The five of us crowded into Dad's four-hundred-square-foot studio in Vallejo, California, with its gigantic disco waterbed and awesome poster of Farrah Fawcett on the opposite wall. We laid out our sleeping bags in the puny living room. The motel-like apartment felt confining, transient, and embarrassing. Back in Minnesota, people lived in houses. Mom and Dad shared the bed, taking advantage of its massive size to sleep as far apart as possible. They had become strange to one another.

For the next seven days, we pretended to be a family. We ate meals together, often at restaurants, and experienced many of the tourist attractions of the Bay Area—most memorably, Ocean Beach and a Six Flags amusement park. We toured unaffordable open homes on sloping hills of the San Francisco Peninsula. Dad's complex maintained a swimming pool. When two-and-a-half-year-old Stevie staggered into the deep end, little hand descending on a piking arm, Dad without hesitation launched from the opposite end and executed an elegant dive that traversed the entire length of the pool. A sputtering and confused Stevie bobbed high above the surface wrapped in his father's arms. "Don't tell Mom."

We were scheduled to fly out of SFO at 8:00 a.m. on Northwest Airlines and arrive in Minneapolis, Minnesota, around 2:00 p.m. We awoke before dawn, ate Raisin Bran out of plastic bowls with mismatched spoons, and made the hour-long drive to SFO, where Dad dumped us on the curb and reminded Mom through the open passenger window to check in with the Northwest skycap before fleeing the scene in an unmarked red Ford Granada. Probably flipped us off. Then we discovered Northwest Airlines had gone on strike, cancelling

all flights. Dense infantry lines of stranded travelers waving
worthless tickets advanced on every service counter. Fathers
at the front. Standing on the busy curbside of San Francisco
International Airport with three squirming young boys, a pile
of luggage, and no clear way of getting home to Minnesota,
Mom looked like a lost little immigrant. Mom put dimes into
payphones and left repeated messages with Dad's office and
on his home answering machine. I don't know whether Dad
received any of these notes or recordings. All we knew was
that he never came back.

Mom took charge. Over the next few hours, the woman afraid of airplanes, airports, contracts, airline personnel
questions, trampling crowds, and public speaking fought her
way to an agent and booked us on another airline to Salt Lake
City, where we had a three-hour layover and enjoyed a free
dinner courtesy of Northwest Airlines before boarding another
plane to the Twin Cities. We arrived at 2:00 a.m., eighteen
hours after another abandonment by Dad. It was dark outside.
But we were not alone in Minnesota. Having tracked Mom's
circumstances all day, Cousin Darlene dispatched two of her
big, burly, smiling sons from nearby Prior Lake to greet us at
the gate and drive us to Darlene's huge home, where four
comfy beds awaited. Safe. There would be no relocation to
California. The marriage would never recover. Over the next
seven years, Dad visited a total of ten weeks, with Mom handling the other 354. The evidence implied we were out of his
mind.

We became one of the first single-parent families to
reside on Northern Heights, divorce being rare enough in the

1970s to be stigmatized with ill-informed projections of adultery, alcoholism, and abuse of all kinds. Broken families usually had to move off across invisible lines into Viking, Valhalla, or Olympic Village apartments. In those days, nice Minnesotans would not say aloud dirty words like "divorce" or answer in good faith the innocent questions of bewildered children, equating such dark-matter language with prurience, blasphemy, or immorality. Nobody talked about such things. Family matters were none of your business. Adding to our confusion, Mom and Dad did not officially divorce until 1978, leaving us in limbo for four more years, confounded and hopeful.

In 1980, Dad hatched a scheme to lure me away from my home, mom, brothers, extended family, and friends. Having researched that Minnesota law allowed children over the age of fourteen to decide which parent to reside with after a divorce, Dad began sprinkling this legality into our phone conversations soon after my thirteenth birthday. That summer, he invited Paul, Stevie, and me to stay with him for two weeks in his new bachelor pad in San Bruno, California. A two-hundred-dollar-a-month, four-hundred-square-foot studio nestled in a massive apartment complex adjacent to Highway 101 where attractive young singles mingled with older, less attractive divorcees. The only children at Shelter Ridge visited on weekends.

We ran around amusement parks, climbed waterslide ramps, stuffed our pieholes with pizza and ice cream, and made regular cart-crashing visits to Safeway, where we picked out whatever we wanted to eat later in front of Dad's

big Sony television: boxes of Banquet chicken and other frozen proteins, pizza disks and rolls, two-liter silos of soda pop,
candy bars, Frosted Flakes, Super Sugar Crisp, and enough
milk to wash it all down. We slept in every day and stayed up
late every night. Forgot to brush our teeth. It was the most
exciting summer of our lives.

The day before we were supposed to fly back to Minnesota, Dad encouraged me to call and ask Mom if we could
stay another month, confiding that he would sell the few
shares of company stock that he retained after the divorce to
keep the good times rolling. We agreed that more was better.
Mom stipulated in a calm voice that masked her pain and legitimate concerns, "Okay, Joe, I want you and your brothers
to spend time with your father—he loves you too." We were
thrilled. A few days after Dad rescheduled our flight home,
Mom learned that he would withhold his two July child support payments, leaving Mom scrambling to pay the August
mortgage.

I turned fourteen that December, and every time I
talked with Dad he would remind me that I was his favorite
son and that we should be together. We did not talk about
Paul and Stevie. By this time, I was a cocky punk with a smart
mouth who had it all figured out. I believed I could con the
con man. Control the dark side. Joey Sith. For the past five
years, I'd envied the kids whose fathers came home from
work and played sports with their sons on weekends. Something in me was so wounded about growing up without a
father that I was unable to care about anyone else. Only me.
The definition of selfish. I blamed Mom. I blamed Dad. I

blamed the world. None of this was my fault. Presented with the chance to have my father back and be loved like other sons were loved by their fathers, I agreed to move to California after the school year. Leave everything behind and start over. Joey Gold Rush. Westward Joey Expansion.

One week before I was supposed to depart, Dad called and told me the big news: he had remarried; my new stepmom's name was Cheri; they had met twenty-one days prior to the wedding; and Dad, Cheri, her daughter, Cindy, and I were about to blend into one big, chunky family smoothie. I thought he was trying to be funny ("Good one, Dad"). Even I knew that adults became engaged before marrying. How could a man who rarely dated and never had a long-term girlfriend be married? How could a man who had fled his family like an arsonist from an orphanage enter into vows with someone other than Mom? What about me? My stumped silence was met with Dad's angry reprimand for not sharing his excitement.

Both my subconscious hopes that my parents might reunite and my fantasy of having exclusive control of Dad's attention and affection were shattered in a single phone call. I hung up, walked into our only bathroom, closed the door, and started to bawl. Mom knocked on the door, came in, and held me for half an hour. Even though my impending move to California was breaking her heart, despite recognizing the pitfalls of me living with an instant stepmother and the disturbed man-child who married her, Mom didn't interfere with my decision to leave. She loved me so much she let me go. I moved to California a week later. Just like him. Joey McDouchebag.

Emerging from the Jetway in San Francisco, I spotted Dad. He was surprisingly pale and orc-like, slovenly dressed with a stupid gap-toothed grin, spindly arm draped around a grimacing, hard-ridden, painted nag who now shared our last name. Compared to Mom's soft, delicate Latina features, Cheri's thickened, yellow, nicotine-infused skin and big bones seemed hideous and unnatural. On the ride home from the airport, Dad gushed like a realtor about Cheri and Cindy and our new home in San Bruno and how I would finally have my own bedroom. But instead of one of the beautiful hillside homes our family had toured in 1975, we pulled up onto a slanted driveway fronting a pale-yellow tract home that resembled a giant cigarette. The surrounding dirt plot was an ashtray of sandy dirt, weeds, and cigarette butts. Losers lived here.

The beige-walled living room showcased Dad's discomforting sofa bed, his technically obsolete nineteen-inch Sony TV, and his high-end Bang & Olufsen stereo system snuggled in a damaged cherrywood cabinet. Stuff even burglars didn't want. No carpets, end tables, plants, artwork, or photos of loved ones—nothing that said *home*. Or *clean*. Or *love*. Dad dead-man-walked me to the entrance of my new bedroom. Nightstand, lamp, and a bed draped with a scavenged blue bedspread cringing with yellow flowers. Hardly the tribute a favorite son would expect. The bedroom I'd left behind in Minnesota had a wooden dresser for my clothes, comic books, matching bedspreads, posters, toys, a stereo, a cedar-filled hamster cage, and a brother. It was like paying with a twenty and accepting change for a ten.

Cheri didn't hate me. Not right away. Needed to give it a few hours. Dad made sure to take me aside that first night, warning with noxious breath, "Don't you ever ask me to choose between the two or you, or you will lose! Do you understand?" Lying in bed that night, I felt cold, tense, suffocated, thick and heavy. A black density sat on my chest. My heart thundered and writhed. My frame shuddered. I was collapsing into myself. I flipped face down and cried so hard that I could hear the bedsprings squeak in support. It felt like the end of my life. I'd never heard of a panic attack.

Dad and Cheri fought like trolls. The two mental patients simmered all day until someone threw some alcohol on that evening's starter argument and they began taking turns snorting language cut with contempt and cruelty. Redheaded Step-Joey became the subject and direct object of countless excited utterances and indictments. Maybe I'd consumed too much milk or generic cereal or left the toilet seat up again. Maybe I needed some clothes or shoes. Or a toothbrush. Apparently, the $250 per month Dad was able to withhold from Mom's child support check based on my residency was not enough to meet my basic needs. I had never felt so expensive. When they ran out of words, one would slam a door. Now it was go time. I'd hear shit breaking. Cheri always escalated to throwing stuff at Dad before marching down the hall to the bathroom, where she'd slam that door. Light up a sniveling cigarette. Dad would run after her, pound the door like a firefighter, and order her to get back to the bedroom. In bad

marriages, the doors and children suffer most. In Mom's
house, I felt safe drifting off to sleep, comforted by Paul reading under the covers by flashlight, the white noise of the
central heating unit, Mom running her bath, The Statler
Brothers playing on the album changer. Nobody ever messed
with our sleep. Not on Mom's watch. Mom always secured
the basics for her children. Now I worried for my safety.
Cheri would stomp down the hallway and burst into my room,
shouting, "I hate you, you little fucker! You ruined my life!"
while slapping me through my bedspread shield. Dad just
stood there. Mute. Moot. Flaccid.

Two months after we arrived in San Bruno, Dad was
reassigned to his company's Santa Rosa office, so we moved
sixty miles north to Sonoma County. My new neighborhood
was a huge improvement: scores of four-bedroom, multiple-
bathroom family homes built around a large high school campus. I met a group of guys on the football field who needed
another player. During the game, two began beating the shit
out of each other as their buddies looked on calmly. Brothers.
Keith Hegarty was two years older, with thin, shoulder-length
blond hair, and wore a white mesh football jersey at least one
size too small, his rockslide arms bare to the shoulders. Dark-
haired Ricky, who was maybe an inch shorter but inches
thicker than Keith, wore a blood-spattered, sleeveless half
shirt revealing steel-cabled muscles. They fought like gladia-
tors. The exchange of "Fuck you, bitch!" signaled a truce and
allowed the game to resume. Keith and especially Ricky, who
years later asked me to be the best man in his wedding, became my protectors and lifelong buddies. Nobody has dared

to beat me up since. And when my home life was too much to handle, their parents, Ron and Debbie Hegarty took me in and allowed me to sleep peacefully under their roof. They loved me like their own son. I learned I could be a happy member of more than one family. I still call Mrs. Hegarty "Mama" and Mr. Hegarty "Pops." Joey Hegarty. Joey Foster.

Three months later, we again piled our crappy life into a rented truck and relocated to less expensive Healdsburg, California, a fifteen-minute drive up Highway 101, where I fell in with some other bored, angry kids with bored, angry older brothers who drove around in pickup trucks to arcades and pizza places looking for trouble. We always found it. I discovered adrenaline and liked it. Rage was a circuit of pain and pleasure. I would throw the first punch and swing until someone pulled me off. Furious Joey could fight all day long. I was hanging out in the high school cafeteria one morning when this guy I didn't know, about my age, came out of nowhere and punched me in the eye. I went WWF on this poor kid and ended up pounding his skull into the cafeteria floor, screaming, "I'm going to kill you, motherfucker!" Two appalled teachers pulled me off. He required a trip to the city hospital. Joey Delinquent was dragged to the principal's office, visited by police officers, questioned by the school psychologist, and ultimately "suspended indefinitely" from Healdsburg High. Something about dysfunctional behavior stemming from unresolved anger and impulse-control issues relating back to traumatic childhood events. I heard TV cop-show terms like assault and battery equated with my conduct. I felt like an asshole.

I sat in my bedroom and waited as Dad handled that evening's phone call. Receiver slam. Shouts. Door slams. Stomping feet. Cheri burst into my bedroom, picked up a piece of ceramic pottery, and threw it at my head. I ducked and sprang out of my bed like I'd discovered a horse head, shrieking, "Don't you ever touch me again!" Cheri lurched away. Dad came at me with red eyes and a raised, milky fist. I channeled my rage, fear, and weight into his white paper chest and launched his unmanly one hundred seventy pounds into the rented wall. "If either of you ever touch me again, I will kill you both! I swear to God!" I shouted. They scurried from my bedroom, gesturing and snarling. I sat on the foot of my bed, my labored breathing hampered by snot and tears. I realized I didn't even know my own father. Joey Skywalker. Biff Joey.

Fifteen minutes later, Dad marched back into my bedroom with the phone in his hummingbird hand. Mom was on the line. Like an angel. Dad hissed into the mouthpiece, "Joe's coming home, Lois." Mom and I cried together like I had just been released from prison.

# Chapter 3

## Prodigal Joey
### (February 1982–July 1983)

Back in Minnesota, I was tackled at the Rochester airport by my tearful family and locked in a seven-month hug, our tiny huddle interrupting the stream of deplaning passengers, tousled and unsteady, blinking eyes scanning for a way out. Mom glowed in her blue winter coat. I sparred and wrestled with an elated Stevie on the way to the frigid car. Paul carried my little blue suitcase. No checked baggage. Malnourished and underweight. Torn clothing and childhood. Cracked shoes, teeth, and eyeglasses. Out of ideas and low on sarcasm. Fragile. Lucky to get out alive. I would complete ninth grade in a well-funded public school system. No reference was made to my assailant loser academic status in Sonoma County, California. Good to be home.

Paul's body and spirit confirmed, to my shrunken horror, that my choice to share Dad's alternative reality had stunted my growth by delaying puberty, that my half year of neglect and trauma stymied research and development of Joey Livermore Labs as time continued to run in a straight line. A life removed from nature. Joey Interrupted. I remembered Paul as a dorky, school-loving bookworm with coke-bottle bottom lenses whom I argued to keep off all of my athletic teams. I used to screw with him, dancing around like Ali, peppering him with fast hands. Push him around. He couldn't lay a hand on me. I had no respect for his physicality.

Now age sixteen and a sophomore at John Marshall High School, Paul had grown two to three inches, had gained ten pounds of dense muscle and bone, and wore a rougher face without eyeglass frames. He'd made the gymnastics team as a still rings and pommel horse specialist, and embraced me in the red leather sleeves of his new varsity jacket: black wool, red trim and buttons, embroidered with a Superman-sized, red letter R. More man than boy. A presence not felt in our home since Dad left. I was pretty sure he could kick my ass. While I had been busy escaping and regressing, the person most like me had chosen courage and progress, reaping well-deserved rewards in a single season. Suddenly, I had a big brother.

Stevie was in the middle of third grade, traversing the steep and pitted childhood mountain trail between helpless little boy and sturdy adolescent. Stevie was remarkably cute from infancy: laughing brown eyes, brussels sprout nose, prominent cheeks, big toothy grin. He sucked his thumb, ran around with a safety-pinned blanket cape, made exuberant Fonzie impersonations, jacked up our toys and comics. He enjoyed the attention of being the baby of the family and of Mom's hypervigilant protection. Got me in a lot of trouble. I loved him so much.

I was reunited with relatives and friends. My doctor, dentist, and optometrist. Fed regular meals. No more beatings. School seemed easier and less painful. But it wasn't long before Mom began telling us about a man named Stan, slipping into her sentences phrases like "been dating," "fallen in love," "has three kids also," and "looking forward to meeting." Another blended family. Sounded dreamy.

Stan was a mechanical engineer at IBM, which in Rochester equated to receiving the Nobel. His eldest child, Stan Jr., was a year older than Paul; his second child, Kirk, was my age; and Katie was two years older than Stevie. All nice kids. Mom's new man enjoyed all of the hypermasculine outdoors activities like hunting, fishing, splitting logs, and DIY home maintenance that my fatherless brothers and I found repugnant and unappealing. Stan made "good money." He was highly educated, held two college degrees, and had completed some doctoral study. He wore sweater vests over short-sleeved dress shirts with pocket protectors. Thick-framed glasses and a full beard. They married on August 12, 1982. We moved into Stan's house and rented out our home on 22nd St.

But there was more to Stan than the likeable nerd. He had lived through an ugly divorce with a hard-living woman who had left him with the children and all of the responsibility. Stan appeared chronically tired and overburdened. While Mom was a faithful Catholic who attended church services religiously, Stan manifested no spiritual underpinnings in his behavior. He had recently recovered from a heavy smoking habit, to which he had devoted decades to sucking back two to three packs of Marlboro Reds every day. Sad people smoke. Unlike Mom's white-glove residence where she scrubbed the floors by hand, laundered clothes every day, and vacuumed obsessively like her device was a dance partner, Stan's large home in Northwest Rochester was as neglected and disheveled as he was.

Mom and Stan committed to constructing a new master bedroom suite over Stan's garage, giving birth to "the Addition." While even the strongest relationships can collapse under the chaos and inconvenience of a home remodeling project, the toddler legs of Mom and Stan's marriage buckled from infinite weighty and thankless duties. During the weekdays, each would put in a long day at work and tend to the avalanche of household work before pounding nails and sanding boards until midnight, leaving no meaningful time for each other or any of the six children. The less hectic weekends allowed for the release of pent-up frustrations and resentments, soul-killing comments, cold silences, and the quiet decisions each inhabitant made to cope in a toxic and hostile environment.

Stan was also a raging alcoholic who consumed hard alcohol like Gatorade. His wet bar in the downstairs family room was occupied by a strike team of half-empty oversized liquor bottles: Smirnoff, Tanqueray, Jack Daniels, Maker's Mark, Jose Cuervo, and Jameson. While both of my parents enjoyed a beer or cocktail when socializing with friends or visiting with family, becoming giggly and gregarious, Stan was an angry drunk who devolved into a braying jackass during his nightly binges. Stan hid much of this behavior during the courtship, employing intellect and humor to address life's challenges, but within weeks of Mom taking his last name, he fell back into the narrative and coping habits of his toxic first marriage: frequent loud, angry tirades; immature acts of passive aggression; pissy, accusatory handwritten notes left on the kitchen table, and a moaning psychological undercurrent of self-pity and cynicism that began eroding the marriage almost immediately.

Unlike any other woman in Rochester married to an IBM engineer, Mom was expected to continue working full-time at the beauty supply store for $3.35 per hour to bring home $100 per week, notwithstanding the fact they had two children in elementary school and an avalanche of household duties required to manage a household of eight people. We should have been able to subsist on Stan's executive take-home pay, Dad's child support contribution, and the income received from renting out our childhood home to complete strangers who shit in our toilet and had sex in our bedrooms. To this day, Stan is the only person ever to disparage Mom's work ethic, openly equating her worth with her hourly wage and the child-rearing responsibilities he devalued and despised, treating her like his minimum-wage caregiver and housekeeper.

Then there was Stan's porn collection. Within the first week of moving into his house, Paul and I located a large, worn cardboard box full of dirty magazines. As though he

wanted us to find them or didn't care if we did. We were familiar with mainstream porno magazines such as Playboy and
Penthouse but grossed out by the vivid and up-close sex depicted in his collection of Yank, Jugs, and Finger. I was aware
and even amused that other fathers hid girlie magazines in
their homes, but never envisioned any of them tossing off to
low-grade snapshots of sad young women while mothers in
the next room folded tiny clothes and stirred meaty casseroles.
Did these periodicals depict how Stan understood women? It
looked like he was making fun of Mom. We were not alone in
recognizing danger signs. Early in the marriage, after observing evidence of abuse for months, Mom's father told Mom to
leave Stan. I love you too, Grandpa.

I focused on school and tried out for the high school
tennis team in my sophomore year. Born with fast reflexes
and exceptional hand-eye coordination and spatial awareness,
I could play any sport. But I was a natural at tennis. Armed
with a 110-mile-per-hour serve and a vicious topspin fore-
hand, unhindered by any formal instruction, work ethic, or
self-awareness, I fire hosed the better-dressed Rochester Tennis Club kids off the luxurious indoor and outdoor courts,
securing through arrogance and brute force one of only seven
available varsity positions. Earned my first athletic letter. My
grades improved dramatically now that I attended all my classes. Anything was better than being home.

Paul and I shared a giant, undulating waterbed in one
of the bomb shelter bedrooms and talked about everything.
Paul disliked Stan, not just for how Stan treated him, but for
how Stan treated his family. We busted each other up making

fun of him. Delivered slowly with Eeyore's dejected expression: "I'm Stan the Man. Moan. Groan. Gloom. Despair. Death." Pantomimed old-man rage and fist-shaking. "The eggshells go into the composter with the corncobs, not in the goddamn garbage can!" I was surprised to see Paul devote so little time to reading. Despite placing in the ninety-eighth percentile on the PSAT in his sophomore year and being solicited by more than a hundred universities, Paul, under Stan's roof, performed below his potential in his junior year coursework and on the SAT and likely torpedoed any chance of a first-rate academic career. It was one thing for Dad and Stan to expect less from Joey Slacker, but I was appalled by the passive-aggressive spectacle of watching both father and stepfather, who earned and benefitted from college degrees, withhold guidance and validation from the most academically inclined member of the family. Seemed like something only small men would do.

The bond between Dad and Stevie was the most fragile due to the open and obvious disinterest Dad had in raising his youngest son. Stevie got the crumbs. Saw Dad maybe five to ten days each year. Chased bounced birthday checks. Suffered long periods of quiet inattention interspersed with cursory phone calls laced with disinterested platitudes. Dad made sure to cut off Stevie's child support six months before he graduated from high school with the memo notation on the check inscribed in his own hand: "Finally." Enough of that.

By the time Stevie was nine years old, his confidence and coping skills had been undermined by a string of personal losses inflicted by obtuse adults without justification or explanation, wounds perpetuated but never acknowledged. He was aware that two men with opportunities to father him had both declined the assignment. Due to our relocation to Northwest Rochester, Stevie was forced to leave the elementary school Paul and I each attended for seven years, starting third grade as the "new student." While Paul and I would graduate from high school and move out in a few years, Stevie would face a nine-year sentence in a halfway house full of strangers, which would force him to rely on a store of stable, life-affirming memories that he did not have. Unable to name his pain, Stevie remained silent. Stevie got lost in all the noise. He was neither an athlete nor an extrovert like me who lived off the social energy of others, or an academic and introvert like Paul who gained sustenance from a life of the mind. His character traits and talents fell somewhere in the middle, his myriad human facets balanced between extremes. He was simply a good kid who liked everyone and whom everyone liked to have around. Stevie just liked to hug people. His state of being, his cool compassion, his virtue of never asking for more than he needed, must have made him easy to miss.

Mom attempted to make up for Dad's indifference over the years by pouring extra love and attention into Stevie's soul, but now, locked into an oppressive schedule and chaotic environment of her own making, Mom was unable to protect Stevie from the natural consequences of such a tragic estrangement dynamic colliding with the toxicity of a crowded, unhappy home led by another indifferent father figure. No logical or loving reason existed to justify Katie and Stevie coming home to an empty house every day after school. But that is what they did.

The following summer, Dad returned to Minnesota for his semi-annual visit. But instead of flying as he had for the past nine years, Dad drove home, which only made financial sense if he was not intending to return alone. Divorced again and looking for company, Dad charmed me into coming back to California with him and promised to send me home on a plane after a couple of weeks. Paul and Stevie were not invited. Dad and I road-tripped to the West Coast like Kerouac and Cassidy, traversing the prairies and mountains of Highway 50—known as the "loneliest road in America"—more in search of escape than any particular goal or destination. When I was little, I often sat on our bathroom counter to watch him tame his morning whiskers just so I could be near him, even for five minutes. Now I had Dad all to myself.

Dad never intended to send me back. Rather, he deployed a brazen campaign of emotional and psychological manipulation more appropriate for a hostage negotiator or a used car salesman than a parent. He promised to buy me contact lenses and a motorcycle without the sweaty inconvenience of attending to the needs of anyone other than myself. I could grow out my hair, buy a leather jacket, skip school, drink beer, and have sex with beautiful girls. He employed every opportunity to remind me of how bad things were back in Rochester, deftly validating my hurt feelings and indignation under the guise of compassion while reconstructing, lie by lie, a vision of an alternative future, one without my mother or brothers, without Minnesota relatives or friends,

without expectations or responsibility, without rules or consequences, without reality or truth, the two of us sharing an
everlasting childhood in sunny Neverland, California. Joey
Pan. Joey Pinocchio the Donkey.

Dad had moved back to Santa Rosa into a low-rent
apartment complex within walking distance of his new office.
He had access to a pool and a Jacuzzi, where Dad would soak
for hours each evening in the company of other middle-aged
underachievers who, like him, had no parenting responsibilities and therefore had ample time to drink beer, smoke
cigarettes, and talk loudly at one another. Dad was greeted
like a celebrity by the inebriated, sunburned hot tub patrons
when he entered the gated pool area in his purple terry cloth
bathrobe. He proudly introduced me to everyone by name before he sauntered up to the picnic table under the pergola,
opened up his portable cooler, and handed me a dew-laced
can of Beck's beer. "I'll bet your mother doesn't allow you to
drink alcohol, huh, Joe?"

"No, Dad." Nor would any fit parent.

The next week was a blur of unadulterated hedonism,
during which I enjoyed the best life had to offer without having to earn any part of it. Like a drug pusher, Dad let out a
little taste for free and promised even more if I was willing to
give our life together one more chance. On the day before I
was scheduled to fly home, Dad and I were soaking in the hot
tub, enjoying a Beck's. Dad donned one of his lying faces and
moved closer.

"Do you really want to go home to your pissy stepfather and siblings?"

Of course I didn't. We skipped debating the reasons for my returning home. Didn't want to get into all that. A few hours later, Dad called Mom, handing me the phone. "Tell her you are going to live with me now."

I remember squeaking into the receiver, "Mom, I'm going to stay here with Dad. He needs me now." Mom's aching sobs pierced through the speaker and were followed by the cries of my brothers. I had abandoned them. Again. My eyes poured hot tears into my mouth. Dad handed me a beer. Joey Deserter. Joey AWOL.

Years later I recognized that Dad's second count of sibling separation stemmed from something more disquieting than loneliness. Any number of people could have filled that void. Rather, Dad hoped my presence would validate him as a parent and therefore improve his cover image as a human being. My father, like the moon, having no light of his own, hoped to shine using the light of a distant son. No matter those left in the dark.

For the remainder of his life, Dad paid a high karmic price for his machinations. My teenage eruptions of violent volcanic activity implied my unconscious was well aware of Dad's duplicity and pathology. During arguments, I got right up in his flounder face and taunted him, glaring, dared him to take his abuse to the next level. Flipped him off. Shredded his diaphanous humanity with rank insults linking him to feces, orifices, and genitalia: ass-face; asshole; dipshit; piece of shit; shithead, shit-face, shit stain, nut sack, dickhead, tiny little prick. I called him Jimbo (his first name is James) in front of people. Told him to go fuck himself. Even when I called him

Dad, my voice squirted sarcasm. No need to take it any further than words. Dad took the metaphorical punches. Usually
agreed with me. He knew what he was.

  The construction project back at Stan's old house outlasted the relationship. Ultimately, expenses outweighed
appreciation, requiring each spouse to take a loss. Without
filing for divorce, Mom left Stan, kicked out our tenants, and
moved back into our childhood home with my wounded
brothers. But it was too late to mitigate Stevie's traumatic
stress. In the dark quiet of Stan's cold basement, either after
school or as six unhappy people found escape in fitful sleep
from shouts, door slams, and prolonged periods of anxious
silence, ten-year-old Stevie consumed his first glass of vodka—an unlistened-for and unheard whisper for help, installing
and activating a time bomb that would lie dormant within the
family for decades.

## Chapter 4

---

## Rise of the Douchebag
(July 1983–1985)

My new life in California began as described in Dad's time-share sales pitch. Without any adults around, I had no adult supervision. Heading out for an evening of traffic violations, illegal drinking, and hanging out with pretty girls, I would make the black-leather-wrapped-astronaut walk across the pool deck to that evening's lineup of hot tub bobbleheads, motorcycle helmet tucked under my arm, and feed Dad the setup line asking what time I should be home. "Twelve, Joe," he would reply. This was followed by a dramatic pause and tired punchline: "Noon tomorrow!" Dad and his fanboys would belch and snort accordingly. And by revving my motorcycle on my way out of the parking lot, I could invoke one final, slurring roar from the plastic cup chlorine people peeing on each other's knees.

I credit Dad for providing the props entitling my horny, curious, wounded animal to roam free—to do whatever the fuck I wanted to do. While I had dated many beautiful fifteen-year-old girls during my sophomore year in Minnesota, none had allowed me to "go all the way." Smart girls. But now I was the easy-riding bad boy: flowing hair and mirrored aviators, angry and self-destructive, the archetypal handsome wiseass ripping wheelies through quiet neighborhoods with one finger in the air. Playing myself in the movie. While most guys won't admit it, they couldn't get laid in high school. Too nice. Too short. Too fat. Too shy. Too stupid. Too smart. But I did. Rapidly and repeatedly. Told everyone. Reason enough to remain in California. It felt really good to be bad. Not sorry. The douchebag always takes more than he needs.

I was reunited with the Hegarty's and my other Santa Rosa friends. "Piner people" represented a diverse swath of blue-collar and short-sleeved white-collar families populating the family-friendly streets in the northwest Apple Tree and Coffey Park neighborhoods, most of whom worked overtime to meet the large mortgage payments that allowed a precarious existence in the very neighborhoods they served. Like Minnesotans, the grown-ups worked hard and devoted leisure time to loved ones, neighbors, and sports. Athletics defined the culture, promoting focused discipline, respect for teamwork and hierarchy, and the overt muscularity required to compete successfully in an economy rewarding only the fast and fit. My buddies were multisport athletes, playing and excelling at varsity football, basketball, baseball, and wrestling. I went out for the tennis team.

I played well enough to earn one of the lower-ranked singles slots and spent the season fending off desperate teammates in weekly challenge matches. I fought for my pride and my school. Won more than I lost. Held my position. A few months later, I was caped in a maroon-and-gold Piner varsity letter jacket like my buddies, my second in as many years. Joey Jockstrap. Wheaties Box Joey. However, while I was building character on the tennis court and in the weight room, I neglected homework assignments, refused to pay attention in class or read books at home, and finally began skipping late-period classes to spend time with my increasing number of dropout friends. When the school administrators reported my unexcused absences and unsatisfactory academic performance to Dad, he ignored them. When my teachers sought an explanation, I charmed them. But when my tennis coach was notified of my inexcusable truancy, I was kicked off the team. Other, less talented but more disciplined teammates—the same guys I beat—would battle for the number-one singles position during what should have been my senior season. I felt like a tool. Still do. Didn't seem to bother Dad.

Paul graduated from high school with a B plus average in June of 1984 and moved out to California with a suitcase, $200, and a disassembled ten-speed bicycle to launch his college career. Dad bought him a bed. Paul and I again shared a bedroom, stoked to be back together. Dad, however, became quickly fixated on creating another "family," of which he could serve as the titular dickhead. Within six weeks of Paul's arrival, Dad moved out of the townhouse he rented for the three of us and moved in with the woman who would become his third wife and abuse victim. This marriage would last three years.

Terry was a polite, intelligent woman in her late thirties, a twice-divorced single mother who worked in ad sales at a local radio station and shared Dad's love of country-western dancing. Her sons, Blake and Dylan, ages fourteen and nine, were both burdened with cumbersome hearing aids and speech impairments. I suspect Terry saw Dad as a source of love and stability based on his children and long-term employment. Meanwhile, in addition to engaging in other behaviors incongruent to a loving relationship, Dad gossiped to his sons and buddies that Terry's face possessed "simian features," comparing his fiancée's face to a primate for a cheap laugh exclusively at her expense. I wish I had told Terry and saved her years of anxiety and grief. Most people step in shit because they didn't see it.

Dad was amused by Dylan, whose age and innocence posed no threat to his authority. But Dad detested the pubescent Blake, referring to his eldest stepson as "Alligator Mouth" (truncated later to "Gator") and initiating a campaign of gratuitous cruelty that included body shaming, mimicking, mocking, and regularly discharging glasses of cold water in Blake's slumbering face to "help" him start his day. Most of this Dad described but never allowed anyone to witness directly, nurturing the possibility that his stories were dark fairy tales as opposed to chilling admissions of child abuse.

Dad's delight in ridiculing weakness or impairment could be traced back to his childhood. Dad shared with his children his greatest hits of misanthropy: denigrating a hearing-impaired nun at his Catholic school by manipulating the volume of his voice so she believed there was something wrong with her hearing aid; tossing to the homeless scalding silver dollars slowly heated with a cigarette lighter; and shooting chickens with a high-powered BB gun so he could enjoy the spectacle of frantic bodies and blasted tetherball heads. While I never believed Dad's apocryphal claim of tying the tails of cats together with twine and throwing them over clothes lines to fight it out, any one of these claims painted a scary portrait of a disfigured soul. Unable to abuse any of his own children directly, Dad found someone else's children to hurt. Paul and I could defend ourselves, but we could not stop him from hurting people.

We were on our own, the apartment crowded every weekend with pretty teenagers, thumping music, alcohol streams, crumpled beer cans leaking tobacco saliva, soiled pizza boxes, and intractable odors. Vanquished carpet, wounded Sheetrock, toxic toilet. But it was not long before Dad, notwithstanding his legal obligation to support me until I graduated from high school in eight months, informed us he was no longer paying rent on the small townhouse for which he had signed a year's lease, requiring us to find jobs and a roommate to meet our bills. Rights do not mean anything unless you can enforce them.

To make rent, Paul got a job at Round Table Pizza and I started working at Big Five Sporting Goods in Coddingtown Plaza. I was now selling athletic sneakers and restringing tennis rackets while flirting with and dating customers and coworkers. It was there that I met a young woman named Cammie, an aspiring model who had a shock of pumpkin-colored hair, green eyes, and a rear end no wider than a ruler. She likely looked good in a bikini. She was always chewing gum. And lucky for me, her recent housing arrangements had fallen apart and she was looking for a roommate. Having nothing else in my brain, I offered to sublet her Dad's upstairs bedroom with a walk-in closet for $125 per month. She accepted. We celebrated at Baskin Robbins, where Cammie polished off a double banana split with four different flavors of ice cream, every sauce and topping, whipped cream, and extra cherries. I remember saying, "Damn, you can eat for such a little girl." She didn't appear to appreciate my consumption compliment. The living arrangement appeared workable the first week, though Cammie quickly drew a line at us stealing her food. She took out her own garbage every day.

Late one morning, I heard a crash from the bathroom. I ran upstairs, put my ear close to the door, and asked if everything was okay. Cammie asked me to come in. The tempered glass shower panel had dislodged from its frame and fallen down on top of her, trapping Cammie like a turtle. I lifted off the door, handed her a towel, and gave her some privacy to dry off, pretending not to notice the fresh legs of pink vomit dogpaddling across the surface of the toilet water, and the spatters of crab bisque clinging to the porcelain lid, tank, and surrounding tile. I heard her cleaning up. Squirt bottle squeezes and bowl flushes. As I helped her reassemble the shower doors, she assured me she was fine. A sour smell nested in my nasal passages for the rest of the day

A few days later when Cammie was out, I was mustard gassed as I passed her bedroom by an odor that implied that something in nature had gone terribly wrong. Joey CSI was on the job. I followed the condensing pungency to the walk-in closet, where it appeared to be emanating from Dad's old garment bag hanging bat-like on a sagging wooden dowel. I pinched the top with my left hand and swiveled my head to suck fresh air before slowly lowering the zipper with my right. Crazy science experiment? Severed pieces of gangrenous ex-boyfriend? Peering inside, I discovered sloshing quarts of stomach slurry fermenting within a piece of luggage that would never again serve its intended purpose. Suppressing my gag reflex, I resealed the giant barf bag, pounded down the stairs, and dragged Paul up to confirm the sighting of what may have been a liquefied ET.

I told everyone the vomit bag story. The next day, a group of us heckled Cammie and her friends as they awkwardly hauled suspicious bags and boxes down the staircase: "Hope someone brought gloves." "Don't spill anything!" More than stupid. Mean. The understanding, compassion, and empathy that I acquired later in life from researching and reflecting upon the fragility and self-destruction tied to eating disorders such as bulimia and anorexia nervosa were not yet available to me. Another reason to go to college.

One of my grandfather's favorite idioms was "He who knoweth not, knoweth not, that he knoweth not." Paul and I savored this embedded sentence, rolling in our heads and mouths the repeating verb, Middle English suffixes, and disorientating triple negative. I enjoyed repeating it to others and feeling superior in the telling, but I began to suspect the *he* in Grandpa's gentle lesson was me.

# Chapter 5

---

## Joey Progressive
### (1985–1989)

My California residency guaranteed my admission to Santa Rosa Junior College (SRJC), a star in the community college constellation that provided quality education and transfer opportunities to the prestigious University of California and California State University systems. A faculty of highly qualified instructors, all possessing master's degrees, many of them with doctorates. Thousands of young ambitious students. I paid the fifty-dollar registration fee and enrolled at the picturesque campus. After my first semester, Terry left Dad and moved back to Montana. Good for her. Paul, and I relocated to Parkridge Apartments, a sprawling, recently constructed complex in northeast Rohnert Park with three pools, two Jacuzzis, fenced tennis courts, and reasonable leases. We rented the second bedroom to a high school buddy of mine who was also attending SRJC. The residents were mostly young adults, students, and evolving taxpayers. Few elderly. Lives in flux. Lives stalled. An island of misfit toys.

There were nine of us at Parkridge enrolled at SRJC, all self-supporting and just a few years out of high school. Eight would eventually earn bachelor's degrees. Our fellowship included Kimmy and Dave, whose wedding I would attend five years later. We remain dear friends to this day. Tall with a mane of dark hair and armed with a sharp intellect, Kimmy was focused on a career in business and finance, intimidating many of her instructors and most of her classmates as she cut down assignments, arguments, and exams. I loved that she didn't take shit from anyone. Dave possessed a quick, creative mind, an infectious energy, and a personality as amiable and gentle as Kimmy's was sharp and intense. He eventually became an architect and a lead guitarist in a local rock band. Nobody was intimidated by Dave.

For one reason or another, each of us had missed the first train to academic success and were somewhat chastened to find ourselves working our way through college hoping to make the next scheduled boarding—the golden admission ticket being the verified maintenance of a B average over twenty courses, requiring approximately three thousand hours of class and commute time, study, and testing. We often met for breakfast at the school cafeteria to talk about our professors and their ideas, failings, and expectations over eggs, French toast (just to hear the cafeteria lady yell out, "FRENCH!"), coffee, and chocolate pudding. We shared stories of family travails and employment duties, comforted by the shared belief that formal education would improve dramatically the quality of our lives. None of us wanted to be left behind. Words flew across the table like Frisbees. We laughed a lot. Played poker for money on weekends. Hung out at the pool. Attended each other's parties.

I signed up for four classes: English Composition, Criminal Science, American History, and Critical Thinking. My professors announced the first day that I was required to show up for every class, read, reflect, and draft my responses to weekly assignments, participate actively in classroom discussions, and acquire enough knowledge over fifteen weeks to submit either a passing essay or pass a test demonstrating my comprehension and ability to apply the acquired theories and concepts to my adult life. They expected me to purchase and carry around fat, floppy "readers," compilations of syllabi, summaries, articles, book excerpts, worksheets, and other hard-copied information in a mountainous backpack that made me look like a virgin. One professor assigned the first five chapters of Jane Austen's Pride and Prejudice and a thousand-word analysis on the dearth of economic opportunities for privileged women in the 1800s. I'll get right on that. Always write about what you know. Another demanded I gag

through long excerpts from Plato's Apology and draft a cogent summary of what I believed to be the common themes.
Wasn't Plato a brand of colored clay putty? What was he so
sorry about? One jackass expected that every submission be
typed. Type this.

Still, this college thing was pretty cool. While high school
required thirty hours of in-person class time each week, my
four courses at SRJC required only twelve hours of roll call
accountability, leaving me 156 hours each week to explore the
limits of legendary sloth. High school girls carried the inconvenience of statutory protections, attentive parents, curfews,
and possible pregnancies, but college women lived in dorms
and small apartments with other college women, practiced
better birth control, and were as eager to taste the pleasures of
adulthood as I was. The first weeks were a blast.

But as the semester and workload progressed, my short-
circuited, limited-storage-capacity mind—devoid of frame-
work, facts, vocabulary, context, and dimensions—crashed
attempting to download so much subject matter. I thought the
word argument meant parents screaming at each other, but my
instructor claimed an argument was a conclusion based on
premises and could be either deductive or inductive. While the
"text" in Pride and Prejudice seemed to be nothing more than
a boring story about oppressed, gold-digging sisters, my English instructor talked about patriarchy, subtext, and irony. My
criminal science instructor talked about a citizen's reasonable

expectation of privacy, which required the government to have probable cause before searching them. I thought the police could do whatever they wanted. I botched pronouns referring to James Joyce and Joyce Kilmer, and confused Shakespeare's Othello with the board game and organic chemistry with good sex. When busted, I owned the dissonance, modeled it like a lampshade, pretended to be a purveyor of fresh-baked puns ("Good one, Joey!"). I wore my ignorance like a toupee. So many of my beliefs and answers were so wrong, so contrary to what actually existed in the world or should have. So much waste. Even sports couldn't save me. I made the SRJC tennis team but found myself outclassed by accomplished student athletes who abstained from sex and keg parties preparing to kick my ass.

I awoke to my lower socioeconomic status and downward trajectory. I saw classmates driving to school in BMWs and Volkswagen Cabriolets who lived on trust funds or "allowances" created by parents with abstract job titles and frequent flyer miles, who traveled to Europe and Asia, spoke other languages, consumed great literature, attended London theater productions, cheered at sporting events in major cities, and developed states of awareness that better prepared them to succeed in a complex world. They were living all of the things I refused to learn. Six semesters and forty-five units later, I made the academic probation list (again). So, I decided not to register for any more classes. Unlike high school, college was voluntary. It was one thing to piss away the secondary educational opportunities legally imposed upon me. But seeing students desperately scribbling their names on waiting lists and sitting on floors of standing-room-only classrooms, I was refluxed over the prospect of displacing students far more likely to benefit from a college education than I ever could. By virtue of not finishing what I started, I acquired my first and only college-related designation: Joey Dropout.

Speaking of losers. Stan wormed his way back into Mom's good graces over a four-year separation. He stopped treating her like shit (or so he promised). Pretended to be less offensive and controlling. Got sober. Converted to a fraudulent, in-name-only Catholicism. Sold his horrible house and moved into a sad, muddy, thin-walled double-wide trailer at Oronoco Estates a few miles out of Rochester. By 1987, Mom had allowed him to settle his intrusive, sick, and decomposing ego into her house on the hill. But unlike Mom, IBM could no longer tolerate keeping an irritable, turgid, vice-ridden, unproductive engineer in its Big Blue family. So, IBM terminated Stan's employment status. Poor Stevie. Forced again to live under the same roof as a proven abusive jerk, Stevie stumbled through middle school into high school. A solid C student. Affable. Popular. Lovable. Class Clown. Too intelligent to fail, but lacking in support to succeed. Stevie learned to drink like a man.

***

Sitting by the pool on a Tuesday afternoon, I noticed a young man across the lot parking in an emerald-green Porsche 911 Targa. As if rehearsed, he sealed the door with a heavy thunk, reached through the open roof, lifted his suit jacket off a wooden hanger, did a 180-degree turn, and walked away from his car buttoning his jacket like John Gotti. Crisp white shirt, pressed slacks, maroon dress shoes with gold buckles. This guy was the male template of everything I believed I wanted to be. I crossed hot asphalt in bare feet to introduce myself and ask him what he did for a living. His name was Lenny. He disclosed that he had graduated from Sonoma State University two years earlier, was credentialed in accounting, and worked as an agent for New York Life.

Lenny got me a meeting with the company's regional sales manager. Joe Bray was in his early forties. Graying hair. Wore suits that shined at the elbows. Radiated patience and kindness. It would take many years before I could appreciate the lack of preparation and sophistication I must have demonstrated during the thirty-minute interview, but somehow I got the job. New York Life Joey, by holding himself out as an agent of the company, was expected to fulfill the ethical and fiduciary duties related to financial planning, master accounting principles and economic concepts, hone oral and written communication skills; and navigate the thatch of federal regulations and state laws governing every operation of the profession.

But the life and disability licensing exam turned out to be an open gate, the level of knowledge expected from the applicant irresponsibly cursory and shallow, similar in depth to the correspondence courses you see in the back of magazines. I passed on the first try, my credential raising expectations of competency I didn't possess. In less than thirty days, with no education or hard-fought credentials, no income or industrial history, no assets, and not a single client, I was ready to peddle financial products as an insurance representative for New York Life with no duty to act in the best interest of my clients. The industry instead relied on the honor system, our contracts demanding that the client assume the risks and burdens of parsing small-font caveat emptor exculpatory clauses that held Joey harmless. I changed my designation to "financial consultant" on my business card because it sounded better. Nobody cared. Could have awarded myself an MBA.

Lenny and I became fast friends and leased a 1600-square-foot house on the tenth tee of Mountain Shadows Golf Course. Rented the third bedroom to Paul. I spent the next eleven months at New York Life pretending to be a financial consultant, earning a decent income and spending my days interacting with honest colleagues and careful clients before novelty transmogrified into drudgery. I had to put on a lot of dance-monkey shows and parrot a lot of canned phrases to convince people born into the middle class to adopt baby-simple fiscal practices and precautions. "Trust me, Margaret, whole life policies are foundational assets in any conservative investment portfolio." "That's right, Mr. Anderson, a well-funded annuity can secure monthly income to last a lifetime." I also couldn't handle the prospect of building a career on a foundation of willful ignorance and the delayed consequences of malpractice in the form of a licensing hearing or lawsuit for gross incompetence. Worse, I was bored. So I quit. Unemployed and subsisting on a $5,000 cash advance at 25 percent interest that would take me years to repay, in a house I could no longer afford, I decided to pursue a career as a stockbroker.

## Chapter 6

---

## Joey Junk Bonds
(1989–1990)

In the late eighties, Oliver Stone released the blockbuster film *Wall Street*, which was based loosely on the celebrated New York City financiers whose convictions for insider trading revealed the pasty underbelly of gross consumerism and immorality permeating the decade. While Stone expected the audience to be repulsed by the malignancy of the financial system and its god-awful characters, Americans celebrated the greed of white-collar criminals, its stars, targets, fixers, posers, philanderers, victims, snitches, prostitutes, and sycophants, who were supported by a society willing to ignore brazen violations of written law and every intangible value America claimed to hold inviolate. Michael Douglas won an Academy Award for his disturbing portrayal of stock speculator Gordon Gekko, a fictional precursor to the legion of self-dealing financial industry shit-bags who thirty years later would exploit federal regulatory loopholes and crater the US economy. I had my new role model.

Lying is more effective when the liar is licensed. Holding oneself out as a stockbroker required passage of the federally administered General Securities Representative Qualification Examination (GS) or Series 7 exam: two hundred fifty questions verifying "the degree to which each candidate possesses the knowledge needed to perform the critical functions of a general securities representative, including sales of corporate securities, variable annuities, direct participation programs, and options and government securities." A Series 7 credential qualified the licensee to trade corporate stocks and bonds, rights, warrants, real estate investment trusts, collateralized mortgage obligations, and a load of other derivative securities. The exam lasted six hours, had no prerequisites, and cost about a hundred dollars. A score of 72 percent was required to pass. The average pass rate is around 65 percent. Far lower for college dropouts. I purchased the Series 7 preparatory material and slogged my way through the definitions, concepts, forms of analysis, terms of art, and federal statutes every professional stockbroker was required to apply when selling corporate equity to the general public. While the abstract legal and financial language made for intimidating reading, it was the mathematics that took me down. Unable to comprehend, much less apply, basic principles of arithmetic, algebra, geometry, probability, and statistics to real life and to other people's money, I failed the valid and reliable assessment metrics of the Series 7 exam. Twice.

The unfit were directed to the consolation game. The Corporate Securities Limited Representative Exam (Series 62) satisfied a FINRA qualification requirement that would allow me to trade corporate securities exclusively. The douchebag loophole. Lower bar of the lesser man. About 86 percent of candidates passed the Series 62 on their first attempt, likely due to the absence of the options/derivatives section requiring aptitude and subject matter mastery of mathematics. I passed on the first try and became licensed. Scored a booster seat on the corporate short bus. Charged some new suits and accessories on a squealing credit card. Off the Rack Joey. Joey Clearance Sale.

I responded to a classified ad and interviewed at Stuart James Investment Bankers in downtown San Francisco, finding myself in a carefully crafted illusion promoting Stuart James's legitimacy in the financial industry: a rapid elevator ride to the seventh floor of 33 New Montgomery Street; a front desk greeting by Jasmine, the nubile, smiling receptionist; preschool-sized gold letters spelling out the company name on the dark wall; copies of *The Wall Street Journal*, *Fortune*, *Forbes*, and *The Economist* laid out accordion style; zests of lemon, lavender, and honeysuckle released by discreet aroma machines. Why would a place this fancy be willing to interview Joey Shortcut? Easy-Way-Out Joey. The company's made-up face implied something to hide.

Jasmine escorted me across the trading floor where well-dressed young men paced, yelling at their phones. Not one was sitting down. I was placed in front of Regional Vice President Jack Kendall, the only guy in the company with a glass-walled office. Jack, his head shiny as a penny, was on the phone, energetically rocking his giant chair and rapping against his desk the spectacular meteorite dominating his left hand. His custom-tailored suit with real buttons on the cuffs hung nearby like a piece of armor. A starched white shirt and sharp collar framed a bright-violet silk tie anchored in a classic Windsor knot. Slamming the phone into its cradle, he banged on the glass wall separating him from the floor. "Get on the fucking phones!" He then ejected from his massive chair and shook my hand like he was running for office.

"Hello, Joseph! Pleasure to meet you!" His grip was firm, powerful.

Jack asked me why I thought I could sell securities. I began disclosing the highlights of my eleven-month tenure at New York Life when Jack cut me off.

"How much did you make this year, Joseph?"

"$30,000, but I have a large commission check coming in . . ."

"You can make $30,000 a month here. Do you want to be rich, Joseph?"

"Goddamn right I do, Jack!" Hallelujah.

We jabbered for a while, but when Jack took another call, I assumed I was being dismissed. Instead, he wrapped his big ring twice on the glass, prompting Jasmine to slip into the office and place a set of documents before me like a hot meal. I was a broker. Joey Bud Fox. Joey Milken Boesky. Jack stood up after his call, seized my hand, looked me straight in the eye, and patted my right cheek.

"I'm going to make you rich, Joseph Dumont. Welcome to Stuart James!" Holy shit!

In 1989, before the internet provided market-monitoring and day-trading tools to the novice investor, stock prices and trajectories were published in a single daily snapshot, divorced from time, motion, and reality. If you wanted to track a stock, you read *The Wall Street Journal* and relied on a licensed professional like me to provide education and guidance over the phone. Honest financial representatives exercise their duties seriously and honorably, seeking in good faith to provide clients with accurate, timely, and legally obtained information. Under this traditional service model, the client's reliance on the broker's advice was based on a long-term relationship of trust and integrity.

My training as a registered representative began the next morning in a small conference room stuffed with wide-eyed, sweaty young men who bragged about degrees in economics and finance from brand-name universities like Michigan, UCLA, and Cal Berkeley. Our trainer, Bobby, an impeccably attired and groomed pitch-weasel who most likely called out his own name during orgasm, slipped into the room and slapped a burly phone list on the table, snarling, "Sit down and shut up!" We did.

"Do I have your fucking attention?" He did.

"Dean Witter, Prudential Securities, and those other nancy-boy investment firms focus only on the big board, the New York Stock Exchange, the NASDAQ!" Bobby announced before pausing a long moment. Then he spoke louder, his tone reflecting disgust.

"Our competitors are corporate cowards. Gutless bed-wetters. Afraid of risk. Afraid of the odds. Afraid of possibili-ties. Afraid of their own fucking shadow! Too scared to make money for their clients. Too scared to feed their fucking fami-lies!" He glared at us. I too began to despise those cowardly companies. Bobby then grinned and opened his arms, transi-tioning to a more inspirational message.

"Here at Stuart James, we're masters of the OTC market. We pioneer financial frontiers. We're the miner-fucking-forty-niners of undiscovered opportunity! We em-brace risk as the engine of all reward. We're players! Welcome to the real game, boys!" I could not wait to get on the phones.

OTC is an acronym for over-the-counter stocks, also known as pink sheets or junk equity. OTCs are banned from the regular exchanges due to problems with valuation, verifi-cation, and volatility. Cash-strapped companies dumped these financial instruments off on investors willing to trade opera-tional liquid capital for infinitesimal equity shares of questionable value. The top-ranked ingredient in an OTC stock is dog shit, with shares selling from pennies to a few bucks—and almost always under five dollars.

Stuart James contracted to unload OTC stock shares related to the initial public offering (IPO) of Cheesy Burrito, a privately held Southern California company. Stuart James's Cheesy Burrito IPO epitomized the speculations of the late '80s, promising quick-flip profits to delusional, middle-aged losers by slapping different labels on lean, long-running fast-food business models traditionally unable to guarantee subsistence to dedicated operators. Taco Bell and Del Taco were already permanent residents of California. Mexican-American family restaurants and food trucks served superior portions of more authentic and higher-quality ethnic and regional specialties every day in every California neighborhood for better prices. Cheesy Burrito never did file its IPO. And the company would flop around like a fish for the next dozen years or so before being consumed by a fast-food franchise for pennies on the dollar.

Stuart James occupied a three-thousand-square-foot space with thick windows and thin carpet, IKEA-cheap furniture, second-rate technology, and a closet-converted glass conference room. Our cage of talking monkeys banging over tables and throwing phones was concealed from public view. The restroom landscape parodied our business model, the single bathroom attracting an all-day reverse-soup-line rotation of thirty young guys, each hauling yards of gurgling intestines as they fought for access to one of only four bathroom stalls. Toilet seats were always oven-warm. Narrow walls resonated butt blasts of Izzy's prime rib marinated in scotch and red wine, and frequent courtesy flushes. Gases and particulates were courageously endured by wincing, misty-eyed colleagues. Encroachments by brokers into bathrooms on other floors were vehemently rebuffed by the property manager, who was forced to field a bevy of complaints from tenants and their clients who resented the smell of shit in the hallways abutting their offices. Assholes.

Jack advised baby-faced brokers to immediately acquire bruising debt. Jack, like the Mob, knew that debt terrified people, creating a motive for immoral or unethical behavior. He encouraged us to take out loans on expensive vehicles we didn't have time to drive, reinvest bonuses into clothing and jewelry we didn't need, drink and dine like paunchy, blood-thickened fifty-year-olds, and lease luxury apartments we would barely decorate and rarely occupy. Jack gave daily shout-outs to the "broker of the day," not for sales figures, but for a broker's recent purchase of a gold ring, Italian suit, or German car. When Tony arrived at work one morning with his hand weighed down by a gigantic Super Bowl ring, Jack treated him like Joe Montana. I felt a deflating sense of pity. Wearing another man's championship ring ranks with wearing another man's Purple Heart medal to show-and-tell. Heroism has never been transferable. I wondered what I could wind up selling to a shaming pawn shop.

I immediately acquired a silky Italian Canali suit, high-thread-count shirts and power ties, and soft Gucci loafers with horse-bit buckles. Some bling. For $900, nearly three times the amount I had ever paid for a month of housing, I leased a six-hundred-square-foot, one-bedroom apartment in Rincon Center's recently completed second tower on the outskirts of the financial district, a massive twenty-three-story building containing a historic post office, commercial office space, and three hundred twenty apartments. A buddy from the firm lived three flights up. Like living in a tree fort. One afternoon after the closing bell, Jack invited us up to The View, a trendy bar capping the new Marriott Hotel on Market Street. Ties loosened, we pounded cocktails, gawked at the dancing lights of San Francisco, and divvied up the world. I

had a blast and a buzz. Jack asked me to pick up the check. I
snapped down my pretty green American Express card. The
bill was $225, twice as much as I had in my checking account.
Equivalent to $800 today. Nearly crapped my new Italian
slacks. Jack forgot to pay me back.

We consummated hit-and-run financial transactions
through faceless one-night stands, exploiting client emotions
and ignorance, cream-filling the informational vacuum with
fabricated statistics, contradictory predictions, creative obfus-
cations, and other damn lies, all employed to pad performance
numbers and commissions *that week*, leaving victims confused, blue-balled, broke, and sore. All legal under federal
law. It took a lot of blurred words to pretty up the corpse of a
decomposing business. We sold confusion. Delusion. Denial.
Latent defects. Saucy shit sandwiches. We called hundreds of
prospects each day with the goal of convincing twenty suckers
to accept our propaganda mailings. Ten received vague rec-
ommendations touting the coming bull market while the other
ten were told tales of the coming bear market. Either way the
market moved, we had hungry fish hooked by our coin-flip
predictions eager to feast on the chum of prior investors. People addicted enough to buy OTC stocks don't need to be
pushed. Gambling, like heroin and sex, sells itself. I became
part of a "fuck you" subculture destined to impregnate and
swell the mainstream over the next thirty years.

A broker cold-calling three hundred people a day is
only as good as his begged, borrowed, and stolen lists of pro-
spective clients. We paid bike messengers fifty bucks to grab
a corporate directory out of the mailroom or impersonated

corporate representatives over the phone to have these lists mailed to our homes. The most-prized directories belonged to insurance conglomerates, big banks, and pharmaceutical giants. We were expected to spin these straw rows of names and numbers into gold. Made my first month's sales quota from a Bank of America directory. When asked how we obtained a private number, we'd own it: "Mr. Johnson, if I can get your private phone number, just imagine what else I can get for you."

We were taught *not* to sell to women: "Never pitch the bitch." Women were too practical to trade OTC stocks, too analytical, too measured. Asked too many questions. A waste of our time. Their relative lack of aggression and unwillingness to listen to our smeary cock-and-ball tactics made them "negative targets." Not surprisingly, few women aspired to work at Stuart James. On the other hand, the silly minds of men, pink brains awash in testosterone, turned to warm, soft putty.

If he said, "I need to talk with my broker about this trade," our response was, "Mr. Johnson, has your broker made you 20 percent on your money this year? No, right? Has he predicted the bull market we're witnessing since our first conversation?"

The client would hem and haw. "Well, no... But..."

"Exactly, Mr. Johnson! Your broker should be apologizing to you for his poor performance. He's an asshole. Probably buying up shares as we speak. Trust me here. We'll start small and go in with only a few thousand. Come on, man. The float is being gobbled up as you finger your marbles. Let's make you some money today!"

We employed "objection stoppers" or "rebuttal files," pre-canned emotional triggers (accurately and hilariously portrayed in *Wall Street* and *Boiler Room)* designed to stitch the deal to the sucker's fat ego. We impressed a false choice: Buy or die. Fuck or walk. Full count. Your move, asshole.

"I just need your social security number to go into trading, Mr. Johnson."

"Whoa there, Joseph. I need to talk to my wife about this."

"Mr. Johnson, do you have a closet in that fancy office of yours?"

"Yeah. Why?"

"I need you to reach in there and grab your backbone. You're making me look like an asshole trying to sell you a used car. I've got a lot more to lose than you do. My reputation is worth more than a lousy five fucking grand!" I would then cue my colleagues in the background to make a bunch of noise: "Joseph, you in? Only ten thousand in the float. Shit or get off the pot!" Men are virgins to a kick in the man-cherries.

After the market closed on a Friday afternoon, several of us, ragged out and punchy, walked down to Jack in the Box to celebrate a shit week over cheap tacos. Some needed release. It started when my new buddy PJ whipped out a gray plastic calculator and requested shout-outs for value estimates of that week's hot companies, prompting a flurry of french fries and smart-ass replies: "Less than I owe in school loans." "Can our answer be less than zero?" "What's 1 percent of nothing?" "Companies?" Laughs and bellows. Sprayed soda and taco meat. Pinch-mouthed, pissed-off patrons. Dark humor is funny, but darkness hides pain. Especially on the inside, where we must have felt the bad we were doing. At some point, the shadows might not wash off. All of us resigned within a few weeks.

Chapter 7

---

## Boston Joey
### (1990–1991)

"What are you doing now that you left Stuart James, Dumont?" Matt asked as he topped off my beer and slid onto my plate another slice of Pinky's pizza. Matt and I met at Santa Rosa Junior College through a nebula of excited new adults who frequented the restaurants and bars on speedy Mendocino Avenue, almost all of whom were able to balance entertainment with disciplined class attendance and prolonged periods of intensive study. We were celebrating his acceptance to Boston University.

"Selling suits at an Italian men's clothing store in Union Square."

"Good times, huh, buddy?" Matt deadpanned. After graduation, Matt would devote himself to learning the language of commercial real estate and eventually take over his father's thriving property company. I, on the other hand, burned down the same academic platform and found myself on my knees center stage in a three-way mirror, running my fingers up the inside seam of wispy Italian fabric that could not shield me from the warmth of another man's inner thigh and hanging plums. Joey the Stitch. Joey Pant Leg.

"Dude! Pack up your shit and move to Boston with me this summer."

Joey Boston. East Coast Joey. I liked the sound of that better. I gestured at cowpath Petaluma Boulevard, remarking dryly, "And what, dude? Leave all this behind?"

Matt sprayed beer out his nose. We toasted over damp napkins. I gave notice the next day. Stored my measuring tape.

I arrived at Logan airport two weeks later with a suitcase. Like a runaway. Matt puttered up to the curb, smiling from his white VW microbus, dressed in the ensemble of tall, handsome, young men coasting along the eastern seaboard and soaring into bright-white futures: wrinkled khaki shorts, faded wrinkled T-shirt, and Birkenstocks. Expertly manipulating the walking-cane stick shift and playground-sized steering wheel, Matt drove us east on 1-90 through the Back Bay into Allston, the "college ghetto": an overpopulated neighborhood of future leaders crammed into winding dominos of brown brick buildings. New images crawled toward and over me as the roadside and memories blurred.

The founding city of Boston channels the grandeur of America's compressed history. Boston is sure of itself. Dignified. Revered. Deeply rooted. Proud harbors. Famous roads. Boston Common, established in 1634, is the oldest city park in the country, born from fifty acres of former cow pastures, surrounded by arbored streets with fabled names: Charles, Tremont, Beacon, Boylston. Three-hundred-year-old churches and brownstones haunt cobblestone streets, housing genera- tions of American spirits who raised our country from infancy. Monuments and structures inspired from classic ar- chitecture of victorious civilizations recast America's intellectual and territorial prosperity and expansion: ornate entryways and arches channeling European castles; tree-sized columns encased in white marble that formerly braced the skies of ancient Greece and Rome; ascending stairways to standing-portrait hallways; heavenly domes and atriums; founding father statuaries. Seemed like an inspirational place to go to school and learn how to make decisions. Or start a revolution.

Matt helped me secure a short-term rented room down the hall from his apartment for $200 per month while the reg- ular occupant was away. He also promised to help me get a job at the course where he had caddied the previous summer. I was a respectable golfer, hitting the links on seventy-one con- secutive days between semesters after discovering men preferred to consummate business intercourse while draining augured holes on manicured mattresses soaked with pesti- cides. I possessed the basic knowledge and technical expertise to advise club selection depending on wind, location, and the golfer's skill level. I spoke Man. Always the subject. But I'd never carried anybody's bags before. Who needed a caddie? They still do that?

Matt picked me up at 5:30 a.m. We stopped for large coffees and glazed donuts at Dunkin before driving ten minutes east past increasingly fabulous suburban estates before Matt made a sudden right turn into the club's entrance. His boggle-eyed headlamps clipped a leprechaun sign: "The Country Club, established AD 1882." Set in a green-and-gray tornado of beautiful trees, Brookline is the oldest country club in the United States, where wrinkled members with sunburned heads pink as penises sip fifteen-dollar lemonades and double whiskies under green awnings on white-beamed porches of the big yellow Colonial-style clubhouse. Shiny green industrial-sized John Deere tractors, trailers, and grooming attachments arranged proudly like toys. Matt parked near the pro shop, and we walked down to the caddy shack, where I was introduced to Danny, who was mustached and middle-aged. Small in Matt's shadow.

"Danny, this is my buddy Joseph. He has a seven handicap and some caddie experience." I had neither. Danny spat a look in my direction.

"If Matt vouches for you, you're good with me. But let me be clear, our members take their games very seriously, and if they tell me you've fucked up in any way, you're gone. Got it?"

"Yes, sir."

"Each loop pulls in fifty to seventy-five dollars. If you do your job right. Got it?"

"Yes, sir."

"Go sit on the hill."

The caddies resembled younger and healthier models of the club's white, onion-skinned members while the darker, smaller humans were not allowed on the course. Except on a tractor. Because Dad's pale, French ethnicity and my Midwestern upbringing dominated Mom's brown, Mexican heritage, I always passed as white, even in Minnesota, receiving the benefit of every racial doubt throughout my life. WASP begins with W for a reason. My face was my resume. I was promoted on my first day.

Brookline members proudly walked these hallowed grounds with their heads held high, knowing they were not like the rest of us. I saw what was going on. Powerful people were attracted to golf. Plenty of custom-made irons and wooden shafts to grip and wave around. Lots of *guy talk*. Ample opportunities for outreach, overreach, and a reach-around. To thrive in this natural habitat, I needed to be one with the bag.

Every douchebag wants to be a big shot. The big hero. His name in giant letters. Mr. Dick Business. Dr. Asshole Spreadsheet. Senator Lance Manhole. I made sure my golfers looked and felt like players. Like the cool kids. Like closers. If we were walking down the course laughing at my jokes and stories, the other golfers could not tell who deserved credit for the comedy. Just two fun guys out having a good time. Fun is good for business because business is boring. Needs a splash of color, some jazz, some Joey WD-40.

I learned to fake deference. While walking the loops, always slightly behind my golfers, I made sure to slip in tactical compliments ("I could hear how well you hit your drive, sir") and Joey-deprecations ("I miss that approach more often than I make it"), frequent follow-up questions ("What do you think you are doing differently based your last three excellent putts?") and extemporaneous expressions of ass-kissing ("You're swinging a big club today, Preston!"). I really wanted these men to like me. And it was not long before Fun Joey was getting loops every Saturday and Sunday, earning between $150 and $200 each weekend.

But in late August: "Dumont! Shanahan twosome at 10:19 a.m." Shit! Dr. Shanahan was infamous for two conspicuous reasons: (1) his more than fifty years of membership; and (2) the afternoon he took a runny dump in the manicured bushes of the back nine before impressing into service a reluctant golf towel to wipe up his rear end—then demanding that the muddy linen continue to dangle off the bag held by the horrified caddie. I had managed to avoid this asshole all summer. But predictably, Dr. Shanahan and I got into it when he insulted my honor after yet another worm-burner into the water late in the round, which merited my clever reminder of his infamous towel's fecal history, prompting the good doctor to beeline it to the caddy shack after he sank his final putt on the eighteenth hole. I did not need to be told I was fired.

***

When the sixty-day lease expired on my rented room, I moved into a five-bedroom basement apartment on Glenville Avenue with a group of cheery new friends. Like the most famous fictional bar in Boston, the windows of the common area were cut six feet from the floor, scrolling frames of disembodied legs scissoring on a treadmill sidewalk. Typical college furniture layered in dust. Old black-and-white television. Industrial metal fan. Budweiser poster. Needed more lamps. Due to the location of my assigned beer-stained futon in the back of the unit, I was dubbed "Sir Joseph of the Hallway" and stored my laundry in a stolen grocery cart often conscripted for beer runs to Marty's corner liquor store.

Chris played The Doors every day. Mike was long and lean and charismatic. They tended bar at the Allston Ale House. V was handsome, hilarious, and hyperspace intelligent, with a dangerous cigarette dangling from his lip that weighed more than he did. Spitz had a smile that could stop an uppercut and always wore Tevas that showed off his thick, hairy feet. Freddy, our mountain man of Chamonix, slept on the least offensive couch and had the rugged good looks of a river guide.

They were college graduates. Sophisticated. Brains woven together with tapestries of scrolled narratives and threads of time. Could quote great literature, offer insights from other cultures, consider laws of science and applied mathematics, inspiring hilarious conversation and insults as they played Nintendo Baseball and took bong hits from Puff the ceramic dragon. They owned precise words for naming the world, categorizing nuances, and balancing interests. Juggled polysyllabic abstract nouns to articulate complex concepts. Employed puns, metaphors, imagery, irony, and sociological context. Comparatively, my worn hand-me-down diction, dangling phrases, and incomplete sentences sounded neglected and shabby. I felt embarrassed about my crappy motel room mind.

The guys roared when a severely hungover V crawled between rooms repeating, "*Metamorphosis!*" and when Freddy's rebuttal referenced a desperate population being "jerked off by Adam Smith's invisible hand." Once, during a debate over Napoleon's attempt to liberate Poland from the rule of Russia, someone made a Polack joke. I didn't get it. Had I simply read the Cliff Notes of Kafka's masterpiece, skimmed the foundational economic theories presented in *Wealth of Nations*, and/or dabbled in the most interesting stories of American history, I could have enjoyed the banter and scored some guy points with my own scorching one-liners. A replaying chorus of Springsteen's "Glory Days" mocked my small, wrinkled bag of powdered high-school stories. My empty sack.

If you don't know who the idiot in the group is, it's you. Without the ability to put the complex sentences of my friends into context, I was shut out. Required to mime laughter or risk damaging exposure. Required to remain silent. Stupid Joey Shut Up. Joey Mumbles. Here I was, holding myself out professionally and personally as some great talker ("The dude's hilarious!"; "You should hear the guy on the phone"). Self-inflicted ignorance wounded my capacity to talk, learn, and even laugh with my own friends. I recalled some of the guys ripping on me: "Read a book, Dumont!" But likely that voice in my memories was my own.

Chris and Mike helped me get me a bouncer job at the Ale House, an Irish dive bar frequented by students from

Boston University, Boston College, and Northeastern, and
even the occasional "overserved" soul from MIT or Harvard.
Ale House customers—offspring of some of the most connected and powerful families in the country, educated at the
finest prep schools on the East Coast, and raised without limits, financial or otherwise—mostly abstained from breaking
house policies and municipal laws. No point in abusing the
hired help. Some flaunted their capital gains through garish
colors and prissy fabrics embroidered with coat of arms em-
blems of decorated institutions. But most chose to wear their
status with rumpled indifference. To act like they had been
there before. I had never disliked so much a group I wanted to
join. I was effective in my runt-liaison role, as most people
who talk bare-knuckled trash are the first to file a lawsuit if
shoved off their pedestals. Most just needed to be talked
down. Recognized. Appreciated. Joey Roadhouse.

A few months later, my Boston roommates moved
away to build marriages and financial security, raise beautiful
children, store happy memories, and create their own dimensions of time and freedom. I flew back to California to live
with Dad.

# Chapter 8

---

## Printed Literacy
### (1991–1992)

Dad appeared gleeful when he picked me up in his bright-red Acura Integra and sped us back to his six-hundred-square-foot, one-bedroom condominium situated behind the Novato Ford dealership. For the tenth move in seventeen years, Dad was accompanied by his time-traveling titanic waterbed, two thousand pounds of bacterial ocean seething inside a rotting frame and decomposing plastic bladder. His poor parenting had the ironic effect of reuniting him with two of his children. Paul's financial position as a student and part-time gymnastics coach required him to bunk on the skeletal sofa bed's tissue-thin mattress and classic debilitating crossbar. His sleep regimen competed actively and unreasonably against Dad's into-the-early-morning television regimen—volume cranked, as if he did not want his son to be well-rested for his fourteen-hour days. Paul spent little time at 303 Mariner Way. I slept side by side with Dad in his waterbed.

Who was I to be critical? Back in Minnesota, only permanently disabled or economically impotent males moved back in with their parents at the age of twenty-four. Even Dad by age twenty-seven had earned a university degree in political science, had celebrated his seventh wedding anniversary, had two healthy children, supported the entire family working as an insurance claims adjuster, owned a home, and drove a new convertible Chevy Corvair. We knew the story well. But in claiming these victories in life's early stage, Dad conveniently left out how the drama ended. The C-average humanities degree that led to a C-average career. Three divorces. A trail of abuse and neglect. Friendless. Alone. Only the dated snapshots mattered to Dad. Never the consequences. Observing Dad bouncing in the driver's seat and enduring a barrage of his vapid, run-together, meandering sentences, I detected something unnatural, almost sinister under the rock of Dad's rapture—a glimmer of triumph.

The perils of my new living arrangements were revealed when Dad, naked as a giant baby, sidled up to the bed at 2 a.m., lifted the bedding, and proceeded to slide his damp ass in next to me, the air pressure of the fluttering sheet generating a gag-inducing waft of his man musk.

"What the fuck, Dad! Put on some pajamas."

"You're not in charge, Joseph."

I sat up and got in his grill. "Listen, asshole, they're called privates for a reason. Normal families wear clothes around one another. I'm not sleeping next to your stinky naked ass. Fuck you!" I glared at him, hoping for the opportunity to smash his simpering face, but Dad immediately waffled as he always did when met with any meaningful resistance. I took Paul's laughter from the next room as a show of solidarity. He liked it when I stood up to Dad.

"Okay, Joseph, whatever you say." He was still scared of me. Glad someone was. What a dick.

*** 

While the internet now serves as a community's job board, glowing with gigabytes of contextually relevant employer listings and serving as an online repository for millions of embellished resumes downloaded and deleted by disappointed employers, job seekers in the early '90s usually reverted to a rudimentary routine of bottom-feeders, scanning the wanted ads with ink-smeared fingers. I spotted a job listing for a sales representative at the Print and Copy Factory, or PCF, located in San Francisco. I figured if I could sell roulette-wheel investment opportunities to timorous poseurs in the casino of penny stocks, I could sell reputable commercial printing and copying services to dynamic Bay Area businesses. Joey the Fudge submitted a resume that may or may not have referenced the award of a bachelor's degree from Sonoma State and was called back for an interview that following Monday.

The morning of my interview, Dad's breath nudged me awake at 7:30 a.m. before he commandeered the toilet for the next half hour, leaving the door wide open so he could share his tips for success between farts and flushes as I shaved a few feet away, resisting the impulse to cut my throat. Once Dad surrendered the bathroom, I showered and put on my favorite stockbroker power suit, an obnoxiously expensive silk tie, and a pair of dark, polished dress shoes that gave me an extra half inch of height before emerging into the living room. Squatting unshaven at the edge of his leather chair at nine o'clock on a Monday morning, casually slurping down a milky bowl of Raisin Bran, Dad sported his pinkish-red terry cloth bathrobe, sans pants, sans underpants, legs wide apart. Nested shrunken apple. He looked up. "You look like a million bucks, Joseph! Who in their right mind wouldn't hire someone so handsome?" I did look good. But Dad's shit-frosted compliment implied my appearance would be the determinative factor in securing this sales position. My friends in California and Boston also looked good in suits, but they brought more than thirty seconds of material to a twenty-minute meeting.

If downtown San Francisco is the girl of your dreams, the industrial basin of San Francisco is her butt-ugly hanger-on cousin from another county. The drive down gunmetal-gray Highway 101 is congested and uninspiring. Concrete overpasses like vampire bats loom above greasy five-lane freeways bisecting the Bay and San Francisco's complex of mills, factories, corrugated metal warehouses, brick chimneys and smokestacks, loading docks, extra-wide roads, trucks and forklifts, miles of chain-link fencing, and Gotham-like fog.

The Print and Copy Factory was housed in a large box of a building surrounded by other randomly sized square and rectangular boxes, as if the city itself had been purchased by

Amazon and converted into a colossal warehouse. The two glass entrance doors were disproportionately small in relation to the factory front, illustrating priorities of containment and security over conditions of access or escape. I was greeted by a smiling young woman and instructed to take a seat. Expansive ceilings, visible ventilation ducts, exposed pipes and insulation materials. The factory walls and floors vibrated with the efforts of unseen machines and operators. My chair buzzed like a tuba.

A few minutes later, a sharply dressed man swaggered up to me and shook my hand. "I'm Gabe Bannon," he said. "Follow me." I was led down a long hallway walled off from factory operations into a bullpen housing twelve desks where six young men, professionally attired and wearing belts holstered with pagers that made them look like gunfighters, paced the room with phone receivers pressed firmly against their ears. Their banter was rapid and emphatic; their voices implied exigency and confidence. The atmosphere was suffused with the same hypermasculine, zero-sum-game competitive energy of Stuart James but without the imbued criminality. I wanted a pager too.

I sat facing Gabe's big desk and my upside-down resume. He slid it away without looking at it. Good start. I bragged about my months of financial expertise, my Series 62 license, and my ability to sell my penny stock shares for thousands of dollars to hundreds of dumb shits until Gabe leaned back in his chair and asked whether I'd noticed the black Porsche 911 Turbo parked at the front of the building. I had. Hard not to notice a high-performance luxury German automobile that approached the price of Dad's condominium. Gabe followed this up by describing his Jaguar and Mercedes as if they were adored offspring. I liked where this interview was going. Two peas in a douche-pod. Gabe and I gibbered like we were on a speed date. Bragged about horsepower and performance handling, low-pro tires and speeding tickets. Our heroics on the commercial battlefield. We talked sports. Gabe offered me a job on the spot selling copies of . . . something. At this point, I was ready to sell myself. Fuller Brush Joey. Joey Amway.

The following Monday, nattily attired—great hair, hands impeccable, clean white collar and Windsor knot, a touch of cologne—I joined three anxious young male sales recruits for a tour of the PCF facility, commencing with the factory floor where I would meet the people who produced what the company wanted me to sell.

Raised in Minnesota where employment is still valued for its own sake, I had developed tremendous respect for physical labels despite my lifelong devotion to their avoidance. Mom's cousins from Prior Lake had operated a family electrician business since before I was born, an economic engine that raised and sustained six children and their progeny. I recall their eldest son acknowledging our arrival one weekend with a friendly wave as he ambled down the driveway with a six-foot, two-hundred-pound water heater balanced on his shoulder like it was a can of Pringles. They came home from work dirty. Hands stained. Obvious muscles. Their "California cousins" seemed fragile by comparison. Paul, who did not complete law school until he was almost thirty-three, took a lot of good-natured ribbing during holiday visits: "So when ya gettin' a job, Paul? You don't get paid reading books, ya know." I was the "pretty boy" who dressed like the bosses and did no actual work.

The factory smells struck first, airborne particles of inks, oils, glues, and solvents laced incongruently with the inviting steam of caramelized bacon and caffeinated coffee beans. Then the mass of its machines. A Heidelberg printing press is as heavy as a school bus, each possessing the gravitas and imperturbability of a steamroller, and PCF had three of them, situated like obese food trucks on wide, clear access lanes demarcated with cautious yellow and hazardous red. Industrial-sized paper cutter blades lifted and dropped like guillotines with terrifying rapidity, precision, and permanence. Glue squirted from the intestines of great binding machines. High-tech photocopiers chirped with the rhythm of crickets.

Function shaped the form of personnel, skill sets, uniforms, and duties. Like the sales team, the print and copy technicians were all men. There were about three dozen or so of them, artisans and supporting cast rhythmically performing choreographed production and maintenance routines, minds meditating on light and vibration, sensitive to any deviation, disharmony, or corruption, as if they had all read *Zen and the Art of Motorcycle Maintenance*. The machinists relied on deep foundations of technical and vocational expertise—compounded by ten-thousand-hour apprentice and journeyman stages until they were recognized by their peers as masters—to manage the rage of the machines. The neckties and long sleeves worn by the salesmen were hazardous to the machinists. Jewelry and multitasking were prohibited for the same reason. Instead, the machinists wore functional clothing, insulating and isolating earplugs and protectors. Safety goggles vs. sunglasses. Lunch boxes instead of expense accounts. They were the artisans, and I would sell their art. I finally felt inspired to hunker down and actually learn something—read something—and actually begin to understand something before I sold it. I was stoked about my new job.

After lunch, Gabe yanked me into his office.

"Enjoying the tour?"

"The factory is amazing. I may have a lot to learn but—"

Gabe cut me off. "I want you to focus on selling copies only."

Was I already being promoted? Gabe could obviously spot talent. What a great company!

"Most paralegals and legal assistants are young women—so you should have no problem making friends," Gabe continued, leaning back in his chair, bright smile widening as he delivered the punchline. "Just don't sleep with all of them!"

"Oh, come on!" blurted my ego. Dad was right. Wrong about most things, but accurate as an atomic clock on this one—I got hired for my appearance, like Greg Brady getting the Johnny Bravo gig because he "fit the suit." Thanks for the nut tap, Gabe. But I was no longer the same person who nine years prior had given two seconds' notice and the middle finger to a Chuck E. Cheese manager demanding I don their choleric rodent costume and allow grade school children rolling on Adderall and Mountain Dew to administer continuous groin kicks. The PCF job duties seemed reasonable and even legal, its people seemed friendly, and the money was good. And I was unemployed and living with Dad.

Two symbiotic elements, love and knowledge, must integrate in any productive interpersonal endeavor. The "love" or process function of my position entailed developing authentic professional relationships with women authorized to contract for PCF services—an insurmountable challenge for a large segment of men, especially those who employ "lines" and "strategies" when "talking up" women as well as the wimps candidly admitting discomfort with relating to half of the world's population. Might want to keep that to yourself, guys. Like children and other vulnerable populations, women are as adept at recognizing affinity and respect as they are at detecting disassembled incompetence and hatred. Women are difficult to con.

The "knowledge" or substantive function of the document management services industry required me to possess working knowledge of every facet of PCF's operation, its culture and vocabulary, its array of products and services, its terms of art, its security, safety, and operational procedures, and the legal duties and liabilities of the company. The learning curve was similar in grade to acquiring proficiency in a foreign language over the weekend. My job was to assess the document management requirements of large companies and law firms and educate potential clients on how PCF's technological and services platform could manage their projects.

PCF competed in a zero-sum game with Knight Rider, a rival company infamous for hiring ambitious salespeople too young to rent automobiles who delivered like Girl Scouts oversized cookies to overworked legal assistants and paralegals in need of a midafternoon sugar rush—a sales tactic I believed dubious until its efficacy was confirmed by every legal assistant I met during my first month on the job. "Can you beat their prices? And do I still get my cookies?" I knew I could do better than cookies.

I commenced a daily reading regimen that I have followed and relied upon to the present day. I began reading industry magazines like *California Lawyer*, *American Lawyer*, and *Stanford Lawyer*, niche publications containing detailed information of civil court filings statewide. I tracked down these firms and began sending the litigators catered lunches. I learned that a term of art assigned a new meaning to a word I thought I already knew. For example, I learned about the vehicles for formal discovery articulated in the California Code of Civil Procedure, the laborious and bulky document production logistics that the services of PCF were designed to address. Testimony came in a variety of forms: deposition transcripts, admissions, forms, and special interrogatories, and most importantly for PCF, costly and imposing disingenuous requests to locate and provide hard copies of every conceivable document, invoice, spreadsheet, and financial statement remotely relevant to the dispute, much of which was already in the possession of the propounding party.

It was through this homework that I stumbled upon toxic tort litigation. And for the record, a tort is not a pastry.

Rather, torts under the law constitute acts of negligence by the defendant that actually and foreseeably cause injury or damage to the plaintiff. You can watch the film *Erin Brokovich* for a reenactment of PG&E's reckless disregard for the lives of local residents and the resulting wrongful death litigation. Or you can visit Flint, Michigan, in real time. Toxic meant poisonous. Poison meant death. Death meant lawsuits. Lawsuits meant documents. Documents meant copies. Copies meant money in Joey's pocket.

Bank of America was acquiring Security Pacific Bank in early 1992, a merger that could keep the PCF machines rolling day and night for the next year or so. So in addition to acting as a bakery bitch-boy to legal assistants to secure relatively modest accounts, I began courting the overpaid associates with newly minted licenses who were forced to sit in cubicles performing "document reviews"—day-long, soul-killing keyword screen searches that are now performed more efficiently and cost-effectively through analytical software. I sent these overworked and disillusioned counselors catered lunches from Max's Deli and hosted happy hours at laughing bars and restaurants within sprinting distance. Not surprisingly, I was awarded the majority of the projects. I loved what I was doing. I learned that engaging in extensive reading and reflection prior to taking decisive action allowed me to evolve like a visiting time-traveler in my new professional arena. Likely for the first time, I had taken the time to put theory into practice, receiving an immediate infusion of moral support, self-worth, and additional income for facilitating a bargained-for exchange benefitting all of the contracting parties. Everyone got what they wanted. All because of me.

# Chapter 9

---

## Transitions
(1992–1993)

While I was in Boston, Paul fell in love with a young woman named Elsa, a recent graduate from USC who stood less than five feet and weighed fewer than one hundred pounds. Paul always got mad when I referred to her as a midget. They got engaged six months later, and soon thereafter, Paul moved in with his fiancée's parents, allowing him to escape the purgatory of Dad's microcondo and focus on his education. I was never a fan of Elsa, and upon learning about her laboratory duties (injecting rats for research purposes), I referred to her as "the Rat" to relatives and even in front of Paul, which predictably inserted a wedge into our relationship. This is what a douchebag does. But she was also smart, ambitious, and a supportive partner as Paul got his life on track. They married two years later. I was the best man.

Dad announced he was moving to Marina Del Rey, a beautiful coastal city just off the 405 near Los Angeles where he would reside for the next ten years. By the early '90s, Dad's policies of taking more than he needed, giving less than the minimum, and shirking all responsibility succeeded in making him obsolete in his own industry. Dad's career as an automobile accident claims adjuster—an insurance professional who interviewed witnesses, took photographs of the scene, produced accident reports, and negotiated liability releases—began with promise in the mid '60s and included a series of promotions and pay increases compounding into the early '80s. But in the final decade of the millennium, the sweeping technological advances in the delivery of insurance services struck like meteors, killing off the walnut-brained, middle-aged dinosaurs unable to adapt to electronic mail, word processing software, and navigating the internet. Consequently, over the next fifteen years, Dad would be fired from a half dozen mid-level administrative positions of declining complexity and compensation in his industry, each more demeaning than the last. He was the West Coast Willy Lowman.

Dad's welcome departure improved my mental health and housing situation, allowing me some much-needed privacy and internal peace. I could afford to take over the monthly $700 mortgage payment on the Mariner Way condominium, enabling Dad to devote his limited resources to meeting his new rental expenses. Dad insisted that he continue to pay the mortgage from his personal account to avoid any "red flags" with the bank and to improve his cratered credit score. Accordingly, the monthly mortgage invoice was forwarded to

Dad's new address. I began sending Dad monthly checks for $700.

In my first year, I became the highest-revenue-producing "copy" salesman at the Print and Copy Factory. My strongest competitor, Mike Birdsall, sold printing exclusively and worked in the cubicle right next to me. He was number one in "printing." While I secured most of my sales contracts sitting across from attractive young women in upscale restaurants or carousing with young associates in liquor-licensed establishments, Mike, tall even on the phone, made major deals based only on the conduit of his voice. He had a phone presence exuding intelligence and optimism, technical mastery and human compassion, and was able to convince from a distance tech companies, hotels, and advertising agencies to contract with PCF.

Mike and I became buddies after he invited me over to meet his wife, Mo (short for Maureen), and their newborn son, Mikey. Mo stood about five feet in heels and had a seven-foot personality and a laser-like intellect. Their son was only a few months old, chubby with saplings of blond hair. He was a stubborn little dude. Thirty minutes after I arrived, Mikey stationed himself in the middle of the living room floor, where he began to hold his breath. Confused, I looked over at Mo, who smiled and whispered, "Just watch." In less than a minute, Mikey began to display various shades of blue while swaying back and forth on his baby blanket before passing out into the arms of his surrounding stuffed animals, causing us to bend over in prolonged hysterical laughter. That was the night I fell in love with the Birdsall family.

Soon after my first anniversary at PCF, I received a call from a former colleague with whom I had worked closely on the Bank of America merger before he was hired away: "Hi, Joseph, it's Tom. I just gave your name to my new boss, Doug Pinter, Executive Vice President of Merrill Corporation, and he wants to talk with you."

"Why me?"

"Doug asked me who the top sales guys were at PCF, so I told him about you and Mike. We have a document division over here that competes with PCF, and they're looking to hire a new sales lead."

My research revealed that Merrill Corporation, head-quartered in my home state of Minnesota, was a publicly traded company that did over $100 million ($100,000,000!) in annual revenue. A week later I received a call from Tom's new boss.

"This is Doug Pinter from Merrill Corporation. I got your name from Tom, and he told me you're 'the man' over there in the copy business."

"All true, Doug. I am quite the copy salesman."

"Would you mind coming downtown to talk with me next Thursday at 2 p.m.?"

As I drove to the interview, I was thrilled to be back in San Francisco's financial district. The Merrill Corporation was housed in a forty-eight-story superstructure at 345 California Street. Stepping off the elevator at the fourteenth floor, I hefted open the thick wooden doors and entered a waiting room. The opulence reminded me of the props employed by

Stuart James in crafting its façade of legitimacy, but I sensed something more substantial beneath the layers of precious metals, fine fabrics, and hand-carved furniture. Waiting for my name to be called, I calmed my nerves by reminding myself I already had a great job. With nothing to lose, I decided to adopt the perineum approach for my upcoming interview: somewhere between dick and asshole.

As I was escorted to the executive suites, I passed a massive, artificially lit mailing room and well-appointed, sunlit conference facilities with sequoia-sized conference tables. Doug was parked in a big leather chair with hawkish views of the city behind him and a wall adorned with degrees and designations, including a law degree from the University of Virginia. He stood up and introduced himself. Svelte and impeccably dressed, with salt-and-pepper hair a bit longer than most executives, Doug possessed a gentility I had yet to encounter in the world of business. No bluster. No mention of cars, money, or where I had purchased my tie. He was genuinely polite. A Southern gentleman.

"I really appreciate you taking time to meet with me, Joseph," he stated, directing me to sit down in a cushioned leather chair in front of his sprawling desk.

We started off with industry small talk, during which I educated Doug on the weaponized gastronomy of copy sales. He smiled the whole time.

"How much are you selling each month, Joseph?"

"Anywhere between $75,000 and $125,000 per month. I acted as the lead on the Bank of America merger."

"You guys sold that work, huh?"

"No . . . I did."

Doug laughed out loud. The ice broken, I switched into my sales persona, rapidly disclosing my base salary, commission structure, bonus compensation, expense account, and every other minute facet of my employment at PCF, sprinkled with reminders that I was "crushing it" just in case Doug forgot. I didn't want the job yet, and it showed. As I prattled on, Doug's fingers danced like a spider across the keys of his desktop calculator before jotting down a few figures on a sheet of paper that he folded before sliding it across the desk. The base salary alone surpassed my entire PCF compensation package. Merrill offered lucrative bonus incentives, a hefty car allowance, a larger expense account, corporate parking in this magnificent building, and a cool new Motorola flip phone (I could be like Captain Kirk). I would let him know my decision by the end of the week. Might have had an erection. Staring at myself in the mirrored elevators on the way down to the parking garage, I looked deranged. I couldn't wait to tell someone.

As luck would have it, Dad was in town on a business trip, so I invited him out to dinner so I could share the news of my career accomplishment in person. I met him at a nice restaurant with large windows overlooking Novato and the surrounding hills. He was waiting in the lobby with a half-empty glass of white zinfandel. Upon seeing me, Dad launched into his "name game," a classic con whereby Dad would memorize and backsplash immediately into any inane restaurant discourse the name of every hostess, server, bar keep, assistant manager, and busboy, an illusory overture promising equanimity and generosity which he would then overleverage by running the entire staff ragged with dainty, insipid requests in exchange for a 5 percent gratuity reluctantly left.

"Joseph, so good to see you. I told Kathy I was waiting for my adult son. Nick, the bartender, even brought me over a big glass of the best wine in Marin County. I told him to put it on the tab. Got my big, handsome successful son to pay."

I thanked the traumatized Kathy and paid Nick for the drink. Dad opened the dinner conversation with "the news dump," tonight's segment an eight-minute exhale during which he described every square inch of his new four-hundred-square-foot studio rental in Marina Del Rey and every new possession purchased on "the credit card." The high-end Trek Mountain bike that would end up permanently parked next to the brand-new forty-two-inch Sony Trinitron television, the postmodern Bang & Olufsen telephone, the handmade cherrywood bedside table impaled with a tall lamp fixture and a small, unstable base, and three hideous art deco pieces of neon-charged glass tubing, one in the shape of a cowboy boot, another a clown. By the time Dad ran out of breath and began slurping his third glass of wine, we had nearly finished dinner.

"Dad, I got the job offer of my life last week!" As I described my new position, salary, benefits, and how excited I was to be working at such an established business organization, Dad, rather than exuding wide-eyed congratulatory enthusiasm, appeared puzzled, his face wrinkling like a pick-le.

"Sounds like a scam, Joseph. Who is going to pay you that kind of money when you have no education or experi-ence?"

"Merrill Corporation, asshole!" I retorted louder than intended, cramming a shiny brochure into his whitefish hand. Should have stuffed it down his large-mouthed throat. "A publicly traded company in the heart of San Francisco with annual revenue over $100 million just offered me a lucrative executive position on its sales team, ass-face!"

"Oh, Joseph, I didn't mean to imply that you're not worth it. I just can't believe they're paying you that much."

I lost my appetite for dessert and paid the check, dis-gusted with myself for expecting my own father to be proud and happy for me. Glances of empathy from the restaurant staff. I thought about pushing Dad down the stairs. The next day, I accepted Merrill's offer, gave notice, and spent the next two weeks saying scores of heartfelt goodbyes to wonderful PCF people. Sometimes you have to give up something good to get something good.

# Chapter 10

---

## Merrill Corporation
### (1993–1996)

The leap from PCF to Merrill Corporation was thrilling and intimidating, fueling the heartburn of impending accountability likely experienced by every minor leaguer called up to the majors. While PCF produced business cards, corporate pamphlets, brochures, transcripts, and bank records, Merrill Corporation printed an evolving business organization's federally mandated compliance publications pursuant to Securities and Exchange Commission regulations, including documents pertaining to initial public offerings (IPOs), mergers and acquisitions, quarterly and annual reporting like 10-Qs and 10-Ks, and prospectuses for dissemination to all of the necessary parties under federal law. Scary adjectives and nouns: mandatory compliance, full disclosure, penalty of perjury.

My next year at Merrill was intoxicating: working aside intelligent professionals in the conference rooms and hallways of top law firms in downtown San Francisco; networking with pretty people at corporate events, conferences, lunches, dinners, and cocktail parties; and getting paid well to learn the intricacies of not only my new industry, but the entire world of commerce and competition. My colleagues and clients included attorneys, paralegals, administrators, compliance analysts, technologists, and senior-level salespeople pulling down million-dollar compensation packages. My terrain changed from bakeries, sandwich shops, and local bars, to fine restaurants, catered reception rooms, and upscale lounges.

My sales colleagues at Merrill oozed confidence compounded by years of disciplined preparation and professional success, but nobody epitomized the Superman archetype more than Paul Hartzell, a six-foot-five-inch man of granite who held a business degree from Lehigh University and formerly pitched for the Minnesota Twins. Like Doug, Paul related to colleagues with social grace, intelligence, humor, and empathy. His golden network of clients included high-level corporate attorneys, venture capitalists, investment bankers, and C-level executives at companies all over the Bay Area.

One sunny afternoon, Paul asked me to accompany him to his daughter's track meet at the Branson School in Marin County. On the drive over, Paul downplayed his professional accomplishments but became very animated when talking about his family life, his still-evolving romance with

his wife, the miracle of raising children, projects he was working on at home, and important friends and relatives in his life.
Paul worked for his family, not just for money or recognition.
In hindsight, Doug and Paul must have recognized I was feeling unmoored and overwhelmed by the powerful currents of
my new ocean and cared enough to remind me that what matters most is the journey home. It was a damn good lesson, but
fifteen years too early.

I decided that if I couldn't match my colleagues with
academic and athletic accomplishments, industrial knowledge,
and high-roller contacts, I could at least dress the part. Breaking the threshold of a nearby Patrick James Clothiers store
with a hot credit card in hand, I found myself in a magical
environment where men in suits were the Mega Men, the
dudes to be adored, accommodated, and served by professional wardrobe designers. Even the mannequins looked like me.
My mood was elevated by a new energy and confidence as I
bathed in images of myself in conference rooms, smartly tailored, posed in moments of decisive action. Like casinos,
clothing stores hide their clocks and crowd the display windows to keep customers focused inward on the carousels and
long wall racks of fine wool suits and slacks, colored cotton
shirts stacked on islands of tables, rainbow waterfalls of silk
neckties, and every accessory necessary to play the game of
the house.

I approached the tailor under a sign that read "Custom
Suits and Shirts" and announced myself. Fred smiled widely,
shook my hand, and offered me a plush leather chair, keeping
to himself the number of times he had performed this same

coronation routine. After some small talk, Fred asked me to step up onto the mirrored pedestal. I was now playing the role of corporate executive, but two years ago I had played Fred on this small stage and could easily reprise this role by popular acclaim. As I remained standing on the dais, watching reflections of Fred bustling around me and chalk-marking my garments from neck to inside seam, I choked up a bit from the complex pairing of pride and humility I felt running down my throat, tasting the hard-won experience that our stations in life are fluid, easily interchangeable, and too often cast by chance. Fred then like an architect guided me over a table of swatch books paginated by obscenely priced fine wool and cotton fabrics for my custom suits and shirts, materials ethereal and soft as suede. Striving to impersonate a Mafia capo, I chose three-piece suits with pinstripes, designing the vests to showcase a newly purchased gold pocket watch. There were high-fabric-count shirts crowned with stiff white collars and French cuff gauntlets, which required the purchase of my first sets of cufflinks. And finally, two pairs of hand-stitched, hand-cobbled Berluti leather shoes. Fred earned a week's commission in a single afternoon. I was suited up and ready to go.

***

I popped out of bed every morning at 5:30 a.m. excited about the events of day, the clothes I would be wearing at these events, and the compliments I would receive about my clothing, before jumping into my detailed RX-7 to run fast and furious down Highway 101. At this level in the corporate world, nobody works nine to five. Rather, in consideration for the huge salary and armored benefits package, an executive is expected to be available, healthy, optimistic, and ready to engage, in person and by phone, every week, Monday through Friday, as early as 7 a.m. for important calls and meetings subject to time zone challenges and to remain continuously available for more meetings, meals, events, and calls until 10 p.m. whenever the situation required. Weekends were more fluid, but the priorities of the employer are written into the rules for every full-time, salaried employee in this country: "and any other duties assigned by the Employer." Nobody called in sick. But at age twenty-six, I was happy to trade the deflated stock of my time and self-worth for a big pot of money and respect.

Flying down the road early one morning, my new cool phone began chirping and buzzing inside my bulky briefcase. Might be a client. I popped open my briefcase, averting my eyes for a fraction of a moment from the roaring freeway to locate my Star Trek flip phone while cresting a hill at seventy-five miles per hour. My brain slammed on the brakes even before my mind had captured a slow-motion snapshot of the stalled pickup truck that was now expanding over my windshield. The sound was so loud that everything went quiet—and fortunately for me, friction outlasted inertia, so instead of having my head sliced off like a cold cut, my beautiful RX-7 Turbo gave its life and engine block to spare mine. A giant straight razor of a bumper rested a few feet from my throat. Two years prior, a dear childhood friend visiting his family one summer between his studies at Oxford and his first year of law school had died in a head-on collision on the narrow farm roads of Bryon, Minnesota, after leaning his long physique into the passenger seat for some unknown reason as he crested the hill in his black VW Beetle. The surviving witness stated he saw neither head nor torso through the approaching windshield. My friend and I made the same mistake. He was buried by his shocked family. I was in the market for a new car.

The next morning in the corporate garage, I saw Doug pull up to the valet station in a glossy black high-end Mercedes Coupe with a black leather interior and sparkling rims. Unlike both of my former bosses, who emerged slowly from the comfortable cabins of their cars, erecting and scanning their surroundings like meerkats for approaching admirers and sycophants, Doug acted like I had just caught him taking a piss, giving me a quick nod and smile as he retrieved his briefcase from the trunk. He handed his heavy car key to Calvin (my favorite valet) and moved purposefully toward the elevator. I decided that Calvin needed a better example of how to own a Mercedes.

It didn't take long to hunt down a classified ad inviting offers on a pre-owned Mercedes Coupe nearly identical to Doug's in Orinda, California. I called up the owner and scheduled an appointment. After the test drive, I handed him the largest check I had ever written and drove home in Doug's car. The next morning, attired in Patrick James's finest and absolutely loving myself, I approached the Mercedes-Benz parked in my garage, pausing a moment to take it all in. I smiled so widely my face hurt. As I sat down in my leather chair, the seatbelt embraced me again, my new morning hug. I pushed a contoured button igniting the sound system, deciding on a jazz station. I bet Doug listened to jazz. Turning onto the Highway 101 south on-ramp, I floored the accelerator, the force of the engine pinning me against my seat as my finely crafted German automobile roared onto the freeway at seventy-five miles an hour, Coltrane blasting from eight speakers. Joey Autobahn. Performance Joey.

But the novelty of playing Doug wore off within a few weeks. The Mercedes was indeed magnificent, but a bit overdressed for the life of a young guy, like wearing a suit to a backyard barbeque. It belonged in the garage of an older man whose life experience enabled him to appreciate the benefits of owning an engine signed by the mechanic who built it, the vehicular equivalent of fine wines and aged spirits. People indeed stared whenever I climbed out of my beautiful car wearing my beautiful clothes, but they did not all appear impressed. Some sets of lips appeared to smile, others to mock. I could have been mistaken.

At a conference at the Hyatt in San Francisco, over four or five drinks, I fostered a relationship with a soon-to-be equity partner at a large law firm in Washington, DC assigned to the AT&T spinoff of Bell Labs. Only in his early thirties, Mark carried the heavy luggage of middle-aged responsibilities, chain-smoking 14 -hour workdays with only a few hours each evening to unwind and enjoy any of the fruits of his labor. And I knew exactly what Mark needed. A couple of weeks later when Mark and his team were back in San Francisco, the four of us dined at Tommy Toy's, one of the most elegant restaurants in the city, its walls adorned with ornate Chinese tapestries and fixtures, the lighting diffused with white candlelit tables. The gourmet Chinese cuisine and sophisticated wine list alone justified my selection, but it was the over-the-top service, three professional waiters assigned like squires and pages to every table, that made Tommy Toy's the perfect venue at which to treat Mark and his colleagues to an experience usually reserved for the richest among us. We drank and dined for hours, laughing our asses off over twenty-dollar pot stickers, Kobe beef medallions, and bottles of fine Sonoma County wines, pampered by soft-spoken servers. As we sipped eighteen-year-old scotch over dessert, Mark and his team awarded his new buddy, Joseph, the entire AT&T project.

Mainlining the endorphin push of this professional and soon-to-be very public victory, I was too excited to sleep that night. Tomorrow would be Talk-about-Joey's-Huge-Sale Day, with all the attention, gratitude, and adulation that successful hunters have always enjoyed, the same emotions, primal and palpable, triggered by the prehistoric cave dwellers who killed saber-toothed tigers. The entire chain of command, even those in our Minnesota HQ, would fixate on the numbers, checking and double-checking the arithmetic destined for spreadsheets, bottom-line calculations, and bonuses. I was huge.

Like a vulture over prey, Dad began circling my life from three hundred miles away. After months of silence, he called almost every day, even while I was at work, paying homage to my newly elevated status and income. "I'm so proud of my handsome, executive son!" he'd say, or "I can't believe how well you've done for yourself." Into this manure-spread, Dad sprinkled seeds of an impending alliance and the financial glory our joint efforts would reap—as if an invitation to partner with a submotivated, increasingly unemployable middle-aged piece of shit was some coveted reward that my efforts had only recently justified. But at the time, I saw the increased attention as a compliment.

I wasn't looking to spend my new windfall, but a week later as I passed by the aptly named Peter Pan Motors, a red Porsche 911 Carrera 4 staged in its center showroom caught my eye. I pulled my Mercedes into guest parking and opened the door, and while I was still seated in my car, a guy walked up to me and said, "Welcome to Peter Pan Motors, sir. My name is Brad. Please let me know if there's anything I can help you with today."

As rehearsed, I emerged slowly from my car, lifting my suit jacket off its wooden hanger, slinging it around my shoulders like Liberace before sliding skillfully into the sleeves.

"Thank you, Peter. You can show me that red 911 in the showroom."

"It would be my pleasure, sir. And by the way, my name is Brad.

The red Porsche had just arrived, a low-mile trade-in from a regular customer who apparently characterized this magnificent racing vehicle as the runt of his litter. I approached respectfully, unlatched the heavy driver's side door, and eased into the seat like it was a hot bath. The tan leather

interior was soft as butter and smelled of honey. When I par-
tially turned the key with my left hand, the dashboard lit up
like a fighter jet cockpit. The oversized speedometer and tachometer, leather-wrapped steering wheel, and video game
gearshift made this performance machine appear almost anxious, frustrated, ready for takeoff. I looked up at Brad.

"Let's take it for a spin."

"Yes, sir."

To accommodate the posturing and preening twenty-
eight-year-old jackass, the staff scurried to move two cars off
the floor to create space for the Porsche to exit the showroom,
capturing the attention of everyone at the dealership. Once the
little red race car was out of the showroom, I jumped into the
driver's seat as Brad began explaining some of its custom features.

"Dude, buckle in," I told him. "We are going for a
ride."

The engine and my heart roared to life when I turned
the ignition. I was in love. As we pulled out of the dealership,
I punched the accelerator. All four tires gripped the hot pavement before slinging three thousand pounds of hot steel and a
pant-shitting Peter Pan salesman down the El Camino Real,
the tachometer needle pole vaulting to red before I power-
shifted into second gear, laughing like a little kid. I tested the
brakes at the next intersection.

"We're taking this thing on the freeway," I announced.

"You break it, you bought it" was the best Brad could
do.

Thirty minutes later, in need of a pit stop, we pulled back into the dealership, the tires smoldering, reeking of rubber cooked in grease, the heat-stroked engine steaming and ticking. A bearded man wearing a long-sleeved dress shirt, tie, cell phone holster, and a sour facial expression—likely Brad's boss—approached.

"Did you have fun . . . sir?"

"So much, I'm taking it home with me."

His face relaxed into a pirate's smile. "Follow me, sir."

The next hour of drama resembled less of an arm's-length, bargained-for exchange and more a hostage negotiation, with my little red Porsche held for ransom by the Peter Pan pirates. I was too emotionally attached to the symbol and my ego to haggle. For my Mercedes, they gave me less than half of what I had paid for it a year earlier. I'm also confident that I paid five figures more to the dealership than the dealership paid to its previous owner a few days earlier for the exact same car. As I pulled out of the dealership, I thought I caught a reflection in my rearview mirror of Brad and his manager high fiving. Joey the Chump. Bent-Over Joey. I noticed a cassette tape in the deck and pushed it in. As I launched my little red rocket onto Highway 101 toward San Francisco, the Bose speakers began to channel Eddie Vedder. I cranked the volume. Like a rock star.

# Chapter 11

---

## The Bar Saga
### (1993–2001)

In February 1999, James David Dumont, age fifty-seven, and Paul Probert Dumont, age thirty-two, would sit for the same California bar exam: Dad in Los Angeles, my brother in Oakland. Whoever passed would be elevated to the status of a licensed attorney, an officer of the court. Esquire. But before I report the verdicts, I'll lay the foundation.

In August of 1993, Dad announced that he'd been accepted at the University of West Los Angeles School of Law (UWLA). I was skeptical about any academic institution willing to stake its reputation on Dad passing the California Bar, the nation's most challenging licensing exam. Period. My research confirmed, however, that UWLA had no reputation to protect. Not in any way. It was not accredited by the American Bar Association. ABA-accredited law school applicants, then and to this day, are required to possess at least one un-

dergraduate degree. Nothing was required from UWLA applicants. Any human being able to qualify for lucrative federal
financial aid gained acceptance. I could have been admitted.
Joey Law.

During Dad's first semester, he invited me to audit his
Real Property class (with his professor's approval of course).
Some of the students appeared new to a classroom. Bored.
Nervous. Overwhelmed. Many appeared to be focused on
their futures for the first time. A few others, like me and Dad,
were simply historic academic underperformers coasting on
currents of laziness, willful ignorance, and entitlement until
their errors and omissions caught up with them in some karmic form, leaving them marginalized, broke, and justifiably
panicked as they crashed through the guard rails of middle
age. Desperation made them delusional.

The uncontested results of this "school" are a stagger-
ing embarrassment. During the decade in which Dad served
his time at UWLA, only 25 percent of its graduates passed the
bar exam. And in February of 2019, only two UWLA graduates passed, while the remaining forty-two failed. A pass rate
of 4 percent. Within the decade, Dad and most of his classmates would default on their student loan obligations, each
with a balance approaching $80,000. In exchange for unim-
proved    circumstances,    hundreds    of    nonperforming,
disillusioned students would suffer long-term emotional, psychological, and financial anguish. Unless they, like Dad, never
intended to pay anything back. Dad laughed at his obligation.
"I got mine, fuck you."

In May 1994, Paul graduated from San Francisco State with a master's degree in English. But he was quickly reminded by the job market that a master's degree was not enough to teach higher ed. And strangely enough, it was Dad who then suggested that Paul apply his love of reading and writing to a legal education to develop more marketable skill sets. Enamored with academics, Paul jumped at the opportunity to spend another four years in school with the ultimate objective of pursuing a full-time position as a legal writing instructor. Paul's admission to ABA-accredited Golden Gate University School of Law in January 1995 put Paul and Dad on a collision course to take the same bar exam. Son vs. father. The pass list is published twice per year on the internet and in every major newspaper in California. The pass rate at the time hovered around 60 to 70 percent; 30 to 40 percent would fail.

For Dad, this match-up violated the axiom that douchebags avoid objective measures of public accountability. Such as a schoolyard fight before an encircling crowd. Or parenting. I couldn't wait to see how it all turned out. If Dad opted out and Paul passed, or Paul passed and Dad failed, the embarrassment of being outperformed on the same professional stage by his own son would be debilitating and permanent, a consequence in direct conflict with Dad's personality disorders. To save face, Dad would at the very least need to make the attempt. If they both failed, Dad could take cover under Paul's disgrace. If they both passed, Dad would bask in the glory of overcoming the most difficult licensing exam in the country with nominal preparation. And if Dad passed and Paul failed, there would be a permanent record implying Dad's superior intellect. So instead of getting off the pot, Dad decided to shit. Because that is what assholes do.

Paul's grades displayed his devotion to the legal profession, earning him some respect for his intellect and the brimming data banks of information acquired through a lifetime of reading. In contrast, Dad adopted the same tactics that expelled him from law school in 1965, ignoring the reading and all other forms of academic engagement. Enrolled in the same curriculum, Dad had trouble passing his exams. But for UWLA's policy of retaining any student able to pay tuition, Dad would have flunked out his first year. Again. He lied about his grades over the phone, claiming to have earned Bs and Cs. I suspect Dad calculated that lack of evidence regarding his preparation would be irrelevant once he passed the bar. To Dad, reward was its own hard work.

Freed up from burdensome reading, critical thinking, and mastering various forms of expository and persuasive writing, Dad began floating the prospect of the two of us opening a civil law mediation practice through which Dad would integrate his skills as a claims adjuster and soon-to-be-licensed attorney to mediate personal injury matters while I would handle the business and marketing responsibilities. Mediation, as opposed to litigation, allows litigants to avoid exacerbating an already-sustained injury (e.g., breached contract; severed limb) with stressful litigation, excruciating delays, exorbitant costs, and a lot of hurt feelings. Mediation is a process wherein disputing parties work closely with a mutually selected, knowledgeable, impartial, and neutral professional, the mediator, who is tasked with dampening the emotions and expectations fueling a conflict by carefully sifting through the objective facts and relevant law to reach a timely, cost-effective, mutually disagreeable solution. The most sought-after mediators were licensed attorneys possessing years of expertise adjudicating and mediating in the specific field of law related to the conflict, as well as the temperament and emotional intelligence expected from a physician caring for a wounded patient.

Unlike most of Dad's fantastical get-rich-quick schemes, this idea had merit. In small doses, Dad could present as charming and articulate, qualities he used to manipulate recently injured automobile accident victims into signing liability releases in exchange for a check of nominal value. Dad made hundreds of tactical in-home visits during which he would plant himself on the couch, warble hospitality requests, and coo honeyed words while maneuvering a pre-printed check before the hapless claimant like a snake charmer: "You can take this check to the bank today, purchase a new color TV, and take it home tonight!" Decades of experience negotiating personal injury and property claims provided Dad with just enough knowledge of tort law and civil procedure to act the role of a successful mediator. All he needed was the black robe of the law to hide behind.

To acquire the experience necessary to open our own mediation practice, Dad logged a lot of volunteer hours between 1995 and 1997 as an insurance claims valuation expert at the Los Angeles Superior Court for a court-sanctioned mediation program dedicated to assisting indigent litigants. Dad was good at resolving small cases with nominal damages. And he was helping people in need (maybe for the first time in his life). These mediations validated the possibilities of our business model. I just needed to get people to pay him for his time. And mine. Sales is easy when you give your products and services away. We decided to open as soon as possible despite our business model being founded on Dad's membership with the California Bar.

Driving to work, I rehearsed versions of my resignation speech, imagining shocked expressions and panicked efforts to talk me out of my decision. But Merrill had a surprise for me. Doug called me into his office.

"Please close the door, Joseph."

Doug broke the news to me that Merrill had lost the AT&T account and showed me the letter he received from Mark that praised my professionalism but eviscerated our Washington, DC office and other sites for failure to communicate and too many incidents of technical incompetence. Doug explained that Merrill intended to restructure some of its divisions and that my position was being eliminated. He looked drained and distraught when he shook my hand. My farewell tour took less than half an hour, the still-employed and unemployed a bit jealous of each other. I would receive my first severance award.

My schedule was now wide open for J. P. Dumont & Company. More on that later. Dad's graduation day from UWLA in June 1997 was comically tragic, a montage of cringeworthy incidents that would have shamed anyone else to suicide. Paul and I drove down for the big event, and Dad's sister flew out with her youngest child from Minnesota. Turned out, Dad was not scheduled to graduate with his classmates after all. His pissy performance on his final exams had dropped his GPA below 2.0. Way to go, dipshit! An administrator explained that Dad could walk with his classmates and receive an empty diploma folder provided he agreed to retake the courses he failed. Rejecting even these shameful accommodations, Dad began to track down and accost each professor who had failed him and beg for a passing grade, in full view of his classmates and their excited families, friends, and camera angles. Out of hearing range but within the zone of embarrassment, we were able to observe Dad's pantomimes of supplication capped off by a gesticulating flourish in our direction: *See, my family is here to watch me graduate!* The facial features and body postures of the ambushed academics evidenced agony of unseen penetrations. We pretended not to know him. Gutless professors and administrators waffled and bumped up his final grades so that Dad could graduate at the bottom of his class. Whatever. As Dad made his grimacing silly-walk across the stage, shit head held high, Paul stuck it to me: "I'm sure he'll do much better on the bar." And then he laughed his ass off.

In May 1998, Paul graduated in the top 15 percent of his class and took the summer off from law, teaching four sections of English at Solano Community College that fall while devoting thirty hours a week to bar prep from September 1998 through February 1999. Dad worked when he could and watched a lot of television. In late January 1999, three weeks before the bar exam, Paul flew down to Marina Del Rey to attend with Dad a three-day MCLE preparation course, an academic emergency mission of mercy he did as a favor to me to help Dad prepare for the multiple-choice section of the bar. This assessment protocol tested capacity for close reading, comprehension of legal doctrines, *and* ability to instantaneously recall the law applicable to a specific fact pattern, at a pace averaging no more than 108 seconds per question. Medical schools use this testing method. Even Paul lacked confidence with the multiple-choice format. Dad presented as supremely confident.

The first day of the MCLE course was dedicated solely to reviewing doctrine for the second day's multiple-choice practice session, which would be given under the same conditions as the bar exam, requiring Paul and Dad to answer correctly at least 144 of 200 multiple-choice questions on six areas of law: contracts, torts, civil procedure, evidence, constitutional law, and property. In fact, the questions used in the training course were more difficult than the questions used on the bar. Participants spent the third day reviewing their previous day's answers. After the second day, I received a call from Paul.

"He didn't finish," Paul reported.

"Could you be a bit more specific?"

"Dad could only get to eighty of a hundred questions each session. He left at least forty questions blank out of two hundred. You can't pass if you can't finish," Paul explained in his teacher's voice.

The bad news came the next day. Dad's raw score was 79 out of 200, while Paul's was 120. Neither would have passed. Paul would spend the next three weeks reviewing multiple-choice questions and answers. No doubt my business partner was doing the same. A week later, I received another call from Paul, who shared with me that he'd left some practice essay exams for Dad to take and mail back for him to critique.

"I just caught Dad cheating on one of the exams. He copied and submitted for my critique the sample answer I mistakenly left with his testing materials. I just spent the last twenty minutes yelling at him."

Dad did not call me that night.

Paul stayed with me in San Francisco all three days of the exam, reporting to me on the last day that he believed he passed. Dad answered the same exam questions and reported the same belief. Three months later, the results were published online after 6 p.m. on a Friday evening. As Paul was coaching, I looked up the results and called him at work to report he had passed. I could hear children cheering in the background. Not surprisingly, James David Dumont was absent from the pass list.

Each received a letter from the Bar: Dad a copy of his rejection letter stating he could pick up copies of his failing exams within a week, and Paul an invitation to participate as a grader on the next bar exam. Dad would take the bar three more times over the next two years, coming close on the second try, but regressing significantly on his remaining attempts before giving up forever in 2001. The relationship between Paul and Dad was never the same. Paul was an attorney, and Dad was still a layperson. To this day, I have tremendous respect for the standards set by the State Bar of California for validating the importance of devoted expertise and for denying Dad his license to steal.

Chapter 12

## Loser
(1996)

The corporate headquarters of J. P. Dumont & Company opened on April 8, 1996, housed on the twenty-fifth floor of the Citicorp building at the corner of Sansome and Market just a few blocks from Merrill. My one-year lease entitled me to a panoply of disembodied office services that depicted my virtual corporation as a thriving business operation teeming with vibrant associates: a physical San Francisco mailing address; an answering and message service ("J. P. Dumont & Company, how may I direct your call?"); access to conference rooms and restroom facilities for my big meetings; and most importantly, a private executive suite for its first president. I donned one of my finest suits for my first day. Favorite shoes, too.

Like a child clinging to a familiar toy on his first day of school, I paid thirty-five dollars to park in the Merrill garage. Laid off from Merrill and burdened by our brassy decision to begin marketing Dad's services before he became a licensed attorney, I felt anxious and unmoored. Even Calvin's reassuring presence was unable to balm the searing fact that I was no longer part of the family. Joey Superfluous. The familiar and comforting sights and sounds of the garage I counted on that morning instead triggered sensations of falling. Enervation. Exhaustion. Nausea. My brain's dimmer switch turned to the lowest setting. The motion picture screen that regularly ran happy movies in my head frayed dark at the edges. A creepy drip of cold sweat channeled down my spine to my butt crack.

I got it together and joined the sidewalk bug trail of workers funneling into the lobby of the Citicorp building to compete for an elevator. Ten passengers. Hairy bike messenger legs tattooed with scars. Some lady's bulky purse pressed into my groin. Someone smelled like a cigarette. I entered the executive lobby and greeted the smiling executive receptionist, taking the opportunity to inform her of my company's grand opening. She looked pretty impressed. "Here is your key, Mr. Dumont. You'll find your office down the hall. It's the third suite on the left." I head-swiveled down the hallway until I saw my suite number. After unlocking the door, I paused for a dramatic moment, my hand on the doorknob, wanting my memory to record for posterity the moment I first entered the executive office of my new company. Big moments made big men. I entered the office and flicked on the light.

My "suite" could not have been more than two hundred square feet. Beige walls without windows or pictures, starved carpeting, four corners shrouded in dusty triangles. Wooden desk. Sleeping phone and table lamp. Slouching office chair. I double-checked the door number. Had I mistakenly leased a walk-in closet? A changing room? Maybe there was a secret door leading to my real corporate headquarters. I felt slashed and deflated. I sat down and pondered my reality. Unemployed. Broke. Unsuccessful scalper of Dad's unlawful legal advice. Peering into the blankness, I understood Dad was not viable. Promises regarding Dad's ability to resolve serious legal matters carried no weight because Dad, like most narcissists, contained no actual substance. Without the weight imbued by a law license, Dad's helium words were not worthy of trust or respect from anxious, greedy litigants, self-interested personal injury attorneys, and burned-out, passive-aggressive insurance counsel. Based on the same premise, neither were mine. I rose slowly from the chair and exited the little room, returned my key to the confused front desk receptionist, and almost galloped to the elevator. Later that afternoon, I called to break my lease, agreed to pay the penalties, and shuttered J. P. Dumont & Company's first corporate office.

A few months later, after we landed our first client in the insurance industry—and after I actually began to believe that we could actually operate a mediation business—I received a phone call.

"Hello, Mr. Dumont. This is Ben Johnson from Sterling Motors. I'm here with your father. He needs you to come down and cosign for his new 750 LI BMW."

"Is that right? Well, Ben, I really appreciate you reaching out to me this afternoon. Would you mind putting my father on the line?"

"Hi, Dad. Ben Johnson tells me you are in the market for a new $80,000 luxury German automobile . . . Are you wearing a straitjacket? Have you lost your fucking mind?"

The little speaker in my phone remained silent. I imagined Dad's contorted facial expressions as he struggled in the presence of his naive and soon-to-be-disappointed new friend Ben to birth a plausible explanation for incurring an exorbitant and gratuitous debt for a creature as despicable and undeserving as he knew himself to be. A few seconds later, he crowned a few words. "I've been working really hard. The payment is only—"

"Tell the salesman you're an asshole!" I interrupted. "Tell Ben you're broke and a liar and that he just wasted two hours on a loser piece of shit who will never purchase a BMW!"

At this point, I would have slammed down the receiver into the cradle, but all I could do was cut the transmission signal of my cell phone with an emphatic thumb gesture. Take *that*, Dad. Then it hit me. The joint savings account. Shit! When we opened the company, we had set aside some cash into a corporate savings account at Union Bank, into which I began making monthly automatic transfers from my checking account. I thought we had enough to keep us both afloat for the next six months. Within a few minutes, I confirmed the available balance was about $500.

A few days later, I felt the STD-like burning shame of finding a formal eviction notice affixed prominently to the outside of my front door. Apparently, Dad stole the mortgage payments I had sent him for the past six months. I ripped the paper off the door like a pee-stained bedsheet, imagined neighbors and delivery people slow-walking past my door and wincing in revulsion or bursting into laughter ("The guy drives a Porsche but can't pay his mortgage! What an ass-hole!"). I shook with indignation over Dad's culpability and from shame over my own. The bank teller told the simple sto-ry over the phone. The bank records indicated withdrawals of increasing frequency and amounts commencing about a year and a half prior and ceasing a few months ago when the ac-count ran out of money. Dad's Wells Fargo records failed to reference any mortgage payments on the Mariner Way condo in the last ninety days. When confronted with the damning evidence, Dad mewled and simpered like a little bitch, de-ploying a scattershot of excuses and deflections, fried-egg face cut up into a grotesque crying yellow smile. I felt like the victim of a crime.

Criminal embezzlement, the act of leveraging one's trusted position (e.g. restaurant manager; father) to deprive and take control of another's property (e.g. that evening's cash revenue; my money), outranks other deprivations of property interest such as larceny because of the added ele-ments of proximity and duplicity; crimes facilitated through betrayals of trust are more unnerving than crimes committed by complete strangers. Stevie once misappropriated and gambled away $3,000 from Mom through cash advances he took out on her Discover card, intercepting the subsequent monthly credit card bills from the mailbox to cover his tracks. The bank was willing to credit Mom's account as long as she filed a criminal complaint against Stevie. Unwilling to risk sending her son to jail, Mom refused.

Therefore, even if Dad's conduct could have been characterized as a crime, the moral implications of reporting him to law enforcement were similarly problematic. Nobody likes a snitch.

Ultimately, Dad's cosigner access to the account combined with my negligence in monitoring Dad's financial transactions put the responsibility back on me. Under California law, my conduct implied a series of gifts or waivers or misunderstandings, creating an atmosphere of reasonable doubt. Dad could simply claim, like he did annually when wrestling with the IRS, that he was an idiot ("I am a pissy money manager!") who thoughtlessly engaged in a series of isolated transactions without any intent to harm anyone but himself. Under the laws of real life, the money was gone and Dad was still my Dad. The warnings Mom and Paul had provided me, lessons learned from their own suffering, were accurate, timely, unequivocal, and made out of love. A pattern was slowly emerging, like twilight stars appearing beyond the setting sun of my ego. Joey Emptor.

I needed cash, so I embarked on a brief but humiliating fundraising tour over the course of which I put the touch on my family and friends for "bridge loans." One buddy mailed me a $10,000 check within the week. Paul maxed out a credit card for a cash advance of $15,000. Then came $10,000 from my Mom and stepfather. Finally, my friend Gary agreed to loan me $10,000. I drove up to Santa Rosa in my shiny red Porsche to take Gary to lunch and collect the funds. With each promise to pay back one of these loans, I could feel an accruing burden of obligation proportionate to the weight of the generosity. I felt like Atlas.

At a stoplight on our way back to Gary's office, I found myself idling next to a Saleen Mustang, a street-legal race car bred for short-term, straight-line acceleration and implanted with an enlarged three-hundred-horsepower steel pacemaker. I looked over to see our counterparts wearing the same idiotic smiles as we revved our engines. I turned back to Gary. "Game on?"

"Dude," he warned, "that's a Saleen. They eat Porsches and shit them out."

Whatever. I threw down the gauntlet by gunning my precisely tuned and perfectly crafted German engine. The other driver responded in kind, abruptly waking an enraged roar from the T. rex trapped beneath his hood. Gary was right. We were about to get eaten. When the light turned green, we popped our clutches, routing the powers of our engines to our drivetrains in a single nut shot. The Mustang launched off the line, accelerating exponentially and appearing smaller with each second. I felt an unfamiliar pop in the linkage of my clutch cable as if my transmission had just blown a hamstring. The torque of the engine overwhelmed the gripping capacity of my low-pro Pirelli performance tires, the scorching friction boiling off rubber in fleshy strips as oily black smoke engulfed the cabin. The driver was polite enough to wait for me at the next light. My embarrassed Porsche hobbled up next to him, smoke and steam hissing from the drivetrain, tires melted like glaciers.

"Had enough?" I asked him. I hoped he peed himself.

The next day, I coaxed my wounded thoroughbred to the nearest dealership. The clutch alone would cost $5,000, the tires a couple more. Numerous other operational irregularities awaited identification and the assignment of four-figure price tags. Broke but needing a vehicle, my only option was to barter a trade-in value sufficient to meet the down payment obligation and back-load any debt by contracting for a longer period of increased monthly payments. I decided not to disclose the prior day's performance challenges, while the dealership staff chose not to disclose anything unsettling about the Range Rover they sold me uncertified at a high markup.

My new pre-owned Range Rover was one of the original SUVs: a muscular engine mounted on a raised chassis, a long wheelbase, and heavy truck tires, all wrapped in a sheath of ivory—a safari vehicle for the jungle streets of Marin County. The expansive cabin, with its broad seats and armrests upholstered in soft, tan leather and interior panels trimmed with walnut, could have accommodated in comfort five NFL linemen. But the appearance of luxury requires constant maintenance, and with no reliable income, I felt I was driving a box of glass into a hailstorm. The Range Rover required a gallon of gas every nine miles. Like the Porsche, its tires and tune-ups ran into the thousands. Insurance coverage in Marin County was exorbitant for such a well-appointed vehicle. There was a hefty annual DMV registration fee. If anything fell off, it was staying off. Hopefully, its previous owner had reported any suspected problems to the dealer when he brought it in.

Wounded and homeless, I began corporate couch surfing at Birdsall Interactive, Mike and Mo's new web development agency. They provided me with my own workspace, the friendship and support of the entire design team, and a safe harbor to pause and reflect on my next moves—everything I needed to keep my frail company and ego on life support. Mo even designed the overall branding concept for J. P. Dumont & Company, including the website, logo, and stationary, a graceful and timely affirmation that my brand had legitimate value. They told me I could pay them back after my company took off. Friendship clarified.

Without enough business to keep my fluttering brain under control, but lonely and increasingly paranoid, I embedded myself like an eccentric relative into the shared lives of the Birdsall family, hanging out at their house three to four times a week, sometimes the entire weekend. Because Mike and Mo's lives revolved around their son, now so did mine. For the next year, I was "Uncle Jofess" to three-year-old Mikey. Mike and Mo must have recognized that quality time with a preschooler was just what I needed. Readers expecting a sensational rendition of child-endangering flubs and mishaps will be disappointed to learn that Uncle Jofess turned out to be a pretty good care provider, notwithstanding my uncontested lack of experience protecting, nurturing, and educating any living children. Safe Sex Joey.

Each morning Mikey would bounce out of bed just after sunrise and lift up the window shade. If the sky was blue, he would turn toward me, holding up the shade like a matador, and announce that day's itinerary: "Happy Day, Jofess. Baseball!" Simple enough. Sunny day equals baseball equals happy. Mikey did not care that I was a loser as long as I could play baseball. I liked these new rules.

I often drove Mikey to preschool, allowing his parents to get to work earlier on demanding projects. As I buckled Mikey into his car seat, I inspected closely the connection of the latches and tension of the straps before defensively driving to Happy Days Preschool. Every time I checked the rearview mirror for his smallness secured in his transportation module like an astronaut, Mikey would smile and wave back, each of us assured of the stable presence of the other. I regularly bought Mikey breakfast with Mo's money at a little Lafayette diner called Millie's. Before he was buckled into his booster chair, Mikey would inform the server, "I want Mickey Mouse pancakes with cherries for da eyes." I often caught myself envisioning fatherhood, imagining one day occupying one of these booths with some dark-haired, fast-talking mini-Joey. Witnessing moments like this changed me forever—a child's innocence spearing the nonsense running through my brain and bringing me back to the present. Then the arrival of the check reminded me I was not entitled to be a father until I could afford to buy my own goddamn pancakes.

The Birdsalls award of parental trust carried the im-
primatur of a public coronation, a validation of my maturity
and value to the tribe beyond my ability to generate commerce
and pay taxes. Like a real adult, I carried my ID to confirm
my vetting and inclusion on Mikey's official list of guardians,
the roster of people authorized to drop off and pick up a student from preschool—one of the greatest honors of my life to
this day. Wee backpack slung over one forearm, colorful water bottle at the ready like a football assistant, encumbered by
stuffed service animals, snacks in airtight containers, wipes,
tissues, adhesive bandages, little shirts and trousers, tiny socks
and underpants, Special Agent-in-Charge Joey was alert and
ready to crash the scene to neutralize all threats to the asset.
Always within arm's reach, I observed every word and action,
stumble and sniffle, and anything within a ten-foot radius that
might do Mikey harm. I inspected his food. I guarded his trips
to the restroom by either entering the stall or positioning myself between him and the public. Head turning, eyes scanning,
I walked him through parking lots and hallways like he was
the president. I began to receive smiles of affirmation from
service providers and even complete strangers throughout
Lafayette. Young women were more likely to give me a second look. Mikey gave me game. I purposely left his car seat
and a couple of stuffed animals in my back seat.

I'll never forget my time with Mikey. Afternoons in
the backyard playing baseball, soccer, and hide-and-seek, digging in the dirt, watching birds and bugs. Dinner served on
durable plastic high-rimmed plates the color of crayons, stub-
by utensils with thickened handles, sippy cups emblazoned

with Scooby-Doo. Fun desserts. Mikey's reluctance about climbing in and then out the bubble bath. The days concluded with the final wind-down: bedtime stories, checking the windows, locating his favorite stuffed animal (a Dalmatian puppy), tucking him into his bunk bed, and switching on the sound machine. His head resting on my chest, damp hair, scent of baby shampoo, and the rhythmic breathing of a sleepy little dude that smelled like bubblegum toothpaste. I never felt such enthusiasm, such certainty, in what I was doing and how I was doing it. I felt my life had a life of its own. This cycle repeated itself at least a hundred times. Thank God. I am indebted to Mike and Mo for recognizing and awakening within me a parenting instinct dormant since childhood, the brief fulfillment of which revealed a much-needed better part of myself when other facets of my life were chaotic and discouraging, and a priceless insight into my own potential to succeed as a father. I'm still working on paying them back.

# Chapter 13

---

## Kimmy
### (1996)

Underemployment is to employment as undernourishment is to nourishment. Alone, downsized, evicted, and owing my best friends and family members over $100,000, I was frightened for the first time in my life—about life. Weakened. Hesitant. Full of dread. For several weeks, no matter how beautiful the morning, I awoke panicked, gasping for air, unable to rise, drowning in the shame of my demoted man-status, deletion from industry networks, and dissipating financial position and career options. Regression, loss, and shrinkage. I sucked. I would lie still. A corpse. Comatose. Try to go back to sleep. I'd hope for unconsciousness. To be someone else. As a result, I slept too long or too little. Sometimes the anxiety surged so hard I'd pop out of bed and walk around in small circles with my fingers fidgeting like I was typing. My mind's terrorized voicemails usually yelled so loudly I thought my neighbors might hear. Something felt infected. Disrupted. Corrupted. The ill in mental illness. Nothing funny about that.

I then began the most impressive emotional eating campaign of my life. Gorging all the same crap I always did when I felt lousy, just more frequently and in ridiculous quantities. For two weeks straight, I binged on sugar-coated cereals. Candy bars. Bloated year-old bean burritos. Crispy packs of sodium-powdered Top Ramen. Stale Cheerios. Lots of delivered Round Table pizza. A family-size Stouffer's lasagna (in one day). An entire thirty-two-ounce block of Tillamook cheddar cheese that I unwrapped like a popsicle. Until gone. Pots of old soup. Orange juice and Diet Coke. Evening pints of ice cream and bathroom sits so long my legs would fall asleep. I gained ten pounds in two weeks. I noticed the emergence of man breasts. Hotdog head. Gooey Nougat Joey. Joey Chubbs. Minnesota Joey Fats. I was a mess.

When life became too difficult, I took the day off and visited Kimmy, one of the founding members of our SRJC breakfast club whose friendship and advice I had trusted and relied upon ever since. Kimmy was a voracious reader, self-educated far beyond her formal credentials, a modern-day intellectual able to critique Faulkner, paraphrase Hawking, and trash Marx in casual conversation. A clear, critical thinker. Long career in finance and wealth management. Anyone who claims to outclass her most likely cannot. But what I believe sets Kimmy apart is her tremendous capacity for active listening and a complementary ability to appreciate and articulate the frailties of the human psyche, dangers of primal impulses, and agonies of existence. Kimmy understands most people better than they understand themselves. Kimmy understands pain.

When she opened the door to her house in Petaluma, I observed her facial expressions shift from placid to alarmed and then concerned as she looked upon the anguished Joey Marshmallow Man crowding her doorstep. Kimmy hugged me, invited me in, and opened a bottle of good Merlot. She unpackaged salty snacks and asked Dave to make some chocolate chip cookies (she knew they were my favorite). I divulged every fact and wound as if a levee had been pierced. Kimmy sat calmly at attention and listened until my reservoir had emptied. She remained present. I heard myself confess, "I would rather have cancer right now than deal with this level of pain."

Kimmy looked right into me. "Wow, honey, you really are a mess."

"I'm breaking," I admitted. "The jig is up. This super confident guy I pretend to be is a fraud, and I'm scared shitless."

Kimmy hugged me, poured me another glass of wine, and slipped a romantic comedy into the VCR. We shared laughter. Fears. Kimmy expressed concern that I'd "off" myself, but I assured her that suicide was off the table. While my uncompromising legislating thoughts were turned against me, my executive branch wanted very much to survive. The collision fused my existential crisis. I was unaware of the human psyche's encased defense installations, such as the mind's pill boxes of denial, deflection, displacement, and sublimation. I had no words, no maps, for any of this. Like running around in a dark room full of dense, shin-level furniture. Roaring in pain.

Kimmy guided me to a number of reference sources on major depressive disorder (MDD), which led to a library of findings of peer-reviewed scientists devoted to understanding this condition. I read for weeks, compared my symptoms, and realized that I did not suffer from prolonged MDD, something more episodic than chronic. Good for me. Like all things toxic, it came down to dosage. MDD is stationed at one extreme edge of the depression continuum, the negative pole of bipolar disorder, the weakest gradation of potential energy within an intelligent organism. MDD is to depression as the Grand Canyon is to a pothole. Read the label. I learned that MDD creates a brownout in the area of the brain that regulates moods and well-being, perspective and problem-solving, locking the sufferer in a debilitating power-saving mode—a precise description of how I had felt for a period of weeks. I recognized the metaphors shared by researchers and literary artists depicting MDD in an eclectic array of isolating barriers imposed on the afflicted: encasing fogs and pitched tunnels, estranging bell jars and long distances, whirlpools and solitary confinement—the suffocating experience of being cut off from light, music, human contact, and other vitalizing sensations of the natural world. Hell of a place to be.

The dissonance between mood and memory imposed by MDD, like physical distance, enables ambivalence, quashes points of reference, and numbs decision-making capacity. The effect was like that on a patient shot with Novocain whose insensitivity endangers the end of his tongue. I learned that mental dissonance at this level alters your ability to make even the easiest of decisions. Action requires a reference point, a beginning. And if nothing matters, there are no distinctions or priorities and therefore there is no capacity to align thoughts, feelings, words, and actions. I found myself staring at the wall for hours on end. Mad at the sun. Absent was my former confidence in my ability to distinguish A and B; it was replaced by hesitancy, paralysis, and confusion. I couldn't focus if I was on fire.

MDD dampens the rehabilitative energies necessary to sustain life. MDD, like AIDS, kills indirectly by disabling an organism's defenses. While AIDS enables previously innocuous infections to become terminal illnesses, MDD disrupts the survivor's coping system and access to positive memories necessary for hope and confidence; stymies regulation of thoughts and emotions based on degree and proportion; and allows despair, hopelessness, agitation, and even thoughts of suicide to rush into the vacuum like a plague. My homework also taught me that our American culture has very little patience with those suffering from depression. Which only exacerbates the anguish of those suffering by imputing weakness, sloth, or some other deficiency of character. So instead of risking being mocked for this newly discovered problem of mine, I decided that I would simply keep this dilemma to myself. The last thing I needed was to be judged as a shameful scourge on our culture. Suicide is preventable, but it demands an act of prevention. Courage. Conviction. Rising action requires handholds of hope. The leverage of optimism. A view of the sky.

The ability to name and conceptualize the facets of my cognitive disruption helped my mind reboot and stabilize, prompting my grinding, lurid thoughts to evaporate after a few weeks. I recognize that part of me was indeed okay with being hit by a truck, or shot by a masked robber at a local bank as I attempted to intervene (I remember this sordid fantasy specifically), but also that this passive desire to die didn't mean I truly wanted out—a clear distinction. I didn't want to kill myself. Thank God for your courage, Kimmy.

# Chapter 14

## Climbing Spirit Joey
### (1996)

Single, underemployed, undereducated, undercapitalized, malnourished, confused, unstable, and out of shape. An oozing cold sore flamed through the skin of my upper lip. Joey Freefall. Joey Rock Bottom. I devoted months to sitting alone, wrapped in silence, pouring over revered texts with cool names like Torah, Talmud, Bhagavad Gita, Qur'an, Tipitaka, Upanishad, and Veda—erudite, scroll-worthy explorations of suffering and enlightenment, compassion, spirit, transcendence, reincarnation, karma, and Tao. I discovered that entire regions of the world play the same game by different rules on different boards, embracing ideologies framed by religions such as Islam, Hinduism, Buddhism, and Judaism. The amelioration of noise, especially my own, enabled my soul to listen patiently to the textual stream of thought and language flowing through my mind. As the weeks passed, my subconscious began generating uplifting images of possibilities, of great spaces far beyond past horizons, first from a distance, then more proximate. I began constructing libraries in my mind. I felt the sculptor of the universe strike off a large section of encasing marble. Schools should cover this stuff. I discovered there were ways of living in this world that contradicted nearly every belief that had informed my perspective of humanity, other curriculums for life founded on stories, concepts, and belief systems I knew nothing about. In Minnesota, if you had time to meditate outside of church services, you had time for more chores or to take on another job. Something about idle hands and devils.

My mind heckled me in Mom's church lady voice as I approached the main doors of the Spirit Rock Meditation Center, a small compound of woody buildings nestled in the pastoral hills of Marin County about an hour's drive north from San Francisco. Small ponds of parking spaces along a winding road bejeweled with shiny, high-end European automobiles, with a few jalopies and classic microbuses interspersed. Kimmy had suggested I explore further avenues of Eastern thought to calm the continuous and compulsive criticisms in my head—all of them arrogant, pissy, and pugnacious, united only in their refusal to go away quietly. I felt like a grenade in search of my pulled pin.

Founded in 1988 and operational to this day, Spirit Rock taught guided insight meditation through a generous offering of residential retreats, seminars, drop-ins, group meditation sessions, literature, and other holistic therapeutic activities such as dharma and yoga. Dharma represents the concept of cosmic law and order permeating Hinduism and Buddhism, while yoga constitutes a group of physical, mental, and spiritual practices designed to put these concepts into human practice, all grounded in Eastern philosophical traditions dating back thousands of years.

I walked into an expansive community room full of people with closed eyes breathing deeply. High ceiling and skylight, white and wood-inlay walls, lots of bare feet and windows, the flooring a reassuring brown-and-orange blanket of crafted finished timber. The air humid with the sandalwood and patchouli oils preferred by hippies and chosen for healing and even aphrodisiac properties. I observed on a small stage decorated with smiling statues a middle-aged man, balding with a robust mustache, gently reminding the gathering to breathe. I sat on a thinning pillow next to people dressed in purple and tried to meditate with my eyes open and then closed. A gracious woman instructed me in the lotus position, an alignment of appendages, pelvis, and spine meant to promote inner attention and free flow of energy. I managed to wishbone my legs into the pretzel position but pissed off my lower back. My mind barked, *This is bullshit! How am I supposed to relax in this dead quiet? My legs are asleep, asshole!* I somehow managed to leave the mediation center feeling more agitated and upset.

On the way home, I stopped at a gas station and inserted my credit card into the pump's electronic reader, expecting its computer to instantly validate my worth to society by authorizing my requested purchase. "DECLINED" appeared in big LED red letters on the digital display. I burst out laughing, tears quickening and rolling down my cheeks. The woman at the next pump began to laugh along with me, but her expression contorted into fright once she calculated she was possibly witnessing a nervous breakdown. I nurtured home my vehicle, ran inside, pillaged couch cushions and pants pockets for dollars and change, and coasted back to the gas station.

As part of my lifesaving regiment, I took up rock climbing as a new hobby, both at indoor climbing gyms as well as on actual cliff faces. Friends asked me, "What do you get out of climbing a wall?" Aside from the carved muscles, cardio benefits, confidence, intellectual stimulation, social interaction, pure enjoyment, and fierce fingers? Rock climbing became my auxiliary mode of meditation and an additional lifeline to its holistic benefits without having to sit on an orange pillow in a room full of people dressed in purple. The other climbers were equally excited to be there and represented a far more diverse and energetic segment of the population than the group at Spirit Rock. They had kind eyes and a relaxed demeanor that matched their clothing—both of which I found comforting. It was easy to strike up conversations with men or women. Someone was always looking for a spotter. Friendly Neighborhood Joey Spiderman.

Indoor climbing gyms usually operated out of large warehouses, allowing the construction of customized climbing walls that present like glaciers or the bows of great ships as high as fifty feet, sections installed at intrepid and intimidating angles and projections. All of the wall surfaces were densely spattered with rainbow-hued rock-climbing holds, shapes molded in plastic or rubber or carved in stone resembling human noses and ears and in numbers so great, the gym walls appeared to be overrun with giant psychedelic bugs. Scores of synthetic belaying ropes hung like rainforest vines from substantial pulleys, bolts, and screws. There is something primal about scaling a wall like a cockroach.

Outdoor climbing required concentrated focus between me and the mountain, allowing an attentive process of aligning the laws of nature (e.g. gravity; inertia) with my body and consciousness to maximize my ability to relate to a massive object numerous stories off the ground. It freed me from myself. I was completely present, my participation undivided and myopic, like I was in a street fight or racing my motorcycle. It was life-changing. When you're leading an outdoor climb, your attention can only be one of two places: the side of the mountain, or oblivion. The cliff or the coffin. When climbing, you notice the friction of your fingers on the granite; your adapted shoes form hooves; hundreds of muscles and tendons throughout the body flex and strain, with never enough recovery time in the long wrestling match with fear and gravity. Sweat beads on the skin, the cooling wind, occasional constrictions of blinding terror—all of these perceptions are primary, present and immediate, without competition or distraction.

Living close to death, time slows down. The edges and seams of life demand an attention capable of blocking out other desperate narratives. Recall the times you have moved close to the edge of a deadly fall from a high position and how you instinctively slowed as the distance between you and the edge decreased, allowing time for weighing the risks of incremental progress. Nobody daydreams on a tightrope. Each climbing performance rehabilitated incrementally my suspect capacity to focus my fiery mind and brimstone emotions, my deteriorating body and big mouth, allowing me over time to experience continuous moments of complete presence and clarity of purpose during my time on the wall, with the added comfort of a safety rope for those moments when my will or execution failed. Through introspection came discipline and accountability. By paying complete attention to my actions, on and off the wall, I began to take responsibility for my own poor decisions and inconsistencies, to root out my own bullshit, and to recognize the needed harmonies of an adult life. As a result, my behaviors became more conscious, more deliberately aligned with nature and spirit.

Arriving at the climbing gym one afternoon with a more buoyant heart and more vibrant imagination, I mistakenly parked in a space zoned for the dry-cleaning store across the street and remained oblivious to my infraction as I gathered my rope and gear from the back of my truck and walked toward the gym. My hearing and peripheral vision captured an unidentified incoming object that my mind recognized as an enraged middle-aged man sprinting out of the launderette, spitting curses and ultimatums, threatening tow trucks and an ass-kicking. Dry Cleaner Guy was closing quickly.

My ego piped up. "Are you talking to me?" At supermoments like this in the past, when I felt threatened, I was the first to jump in, get the first shot in, and pummel until someone pulled me off. But my current mood overruled my historical reaction to possible violence. My recent homework had also taught me that now was a good time to be present for this man, to acknowledge his spirit and leave my ego behind. He needed to matter as much as me. I stood still, arms down, gathered my courage, and simply observed him as he slowed his approach toward me. At the existential level, I knew this dude. He was a mess, too. And he felt aggrieved, shit upon and disrespected by the world, just like I had felt lately, and he believed I had purposely ignored his clearly demarcated public sign—which required him to yet again anxiously confront a stranger too rude to follow the laws of a polite society. I could add to or alleviate his suffering. I squared my body to face him like a mirror, looked into his puffing face, relaxed the muscles of my own body, smiled, and said, "Oh man, I'm sorry. I was lost in thought and excited to get on the wall. I'll move it right away."

The man's angry energy deflated like a dying balloon, leaving him limp and confused. I had responded without judgment, malice, or anger, and most importantly, without fear. My apology was genuine, and he got that. The man recovered himself. "No . . . I'm sorry . . . Go ahead and leave it there, young man, and have a good climb."

I smiled. "I will, sir, and thanks!"

# Chapter 15

## Joey Beaujolais
(1997)

Working through a stack of outraged mail ("delinquent"; "final notice"; "notice of collection"; "notice of fuck you"), each envelope disclosing another rotting account balance, oppressive late penalty, exorbitant interest charge, and polite reminder of the ramifications of collection litigation and an adverse credit history, I noticed a triangle of powder blue paper peeking out of the leaning deck of white envelopes. A birthday card with stickers of kittens and my name spelled out in Mom's impeccable, flowing cursive script. She had written on the inside, "Happy Birthday, Joe. I love you and we are very proud of you. Love, Mom, Stan, and Sammy." Sammy was her cat. A check imprinted with kitten photos and made out for fifty dollars slid out, "For Pizza" handwritten in the memo section. I was still her little boy after thirty-one years. I cried like a man.

It was a beautiful day, seventy degrees in December, clear sky. I decided to enjoy the walk over to Bank of America to deposit my new windfall. Smell some roses. Seize the day. That kind of thing. On the way out, I noticed my white Range Rover leaning starboard as if hip-checked by an iceberg. On closer inspection, each passenger-side tire had suffered multiple stab wounds. "Rich Prick" was etched onto the dusty mural of my back cargo window by a vandal's filthy index finger. I had to sit down. Take the mandatory standing eight count. I got back up. I called AAA and had my truck towed to a tire service shop: "Yes, it is a beautiful day. So you're saying all four require replacement. Estimate of $1,000? Great! You take credit cards, right?"

After depositing Mom's check, I bought a newspaper and occupied an outdoor table of a San Francisco coffee shop to review the classifieds. Each posting contained disqualifying phrases such as "prerequisites," "bachelor's degree," and "mandatory experience." Random anxious memories. Confidence is another name for spirit, and mine was as deflated as my tires. A parachute aerated by a thousand cuts. Sweet moments of human contact—the draught and sustenance of society, the extrovert's elixir— tasted bitter when tainted with my broken promises, preventable errors, and shamed ego. I suffered through calls negotiating delinquent account balances and apologies with investors. Closed our overdrawn corporate accounts in front of an embarrassed banker. Slogged through endless takes of exhausting internal monologues, cuts and scraps rough and heavy as shingles. I believed my present state of mind would expose me to more ridicule than my high school diploma would in attempting immediate reentry into the atmosphere of corporate sales. If I was wrong about all this, I had no way of telling the difference.

So I did what most men would do when confronted with a crisis of confidence.

"Hi, Mom. I'm a mess." I reported Dad's fiduciary breaches of trust and outright thievery, his indifference toward his legal training and ethical standards, his pathologies likely to harm business partners and potential clients. I shared that our business venture had failed, completely and finally. I acknowledged my own contributions to my demise. Finally, I disclosed the marathon raves thumping in my mind's empty warehouse, the gushers of stomach acid, and the dark headaches that sprang in broad daylight that would keep me out of commission for a while.

"Oh, honey, why don't you come home and stay with your old mom?"

"I appreciate the offer, but I can't fix my adult life from my childhood bedroom."

"Well, what are you going to do then, Joe?"

"I have no idea, Mom. That's why I'm calling you."

She laughed, then paused for a moment before observing, "Why don't you get a job as a waiter again? You made darn good money doing that in college." To Mom, "darn good money" was more than ten dollars per hour.

"Well, Mom, for starters I owe over $100,000 to you and my friends."

"You need to eat first and worry about the big bills later. Both your brothers are working jobs earning fifteen dollars per hour. One day at a time. Remember how Pat Braunhausen sang that song so beautifully at your Grandmother's funeral?" I did. After we ended the call, I updated my resume. Somehow my unannounced arrival at Zingari Ristorante in San Francisco's Union Square, lack of professional experience, and impromptu interview with Kristian the owner got me hired as a server. I drove home and called Mom. I felt proud of myself. From clods of manure grew saplings of hope.

I probably should have memorized the culinary descriptions and prices printed in Zingari's menu, conducted some research on the ingredients and preparation of each offered item, and engaged in a similar process of research and reflection regarding Zingari's sophisticated wine list and full bar. Instead, I showed up for my first training shift oblivious and unprepared, much to the disappointment of Executive Chef Cameron, who conveyed his displeasure through a passionate tirade of expletives and insults mostly reserved for Kristian and his mother.

Chef Cameron took me back to the kitchen and introduced me to other chefs, servers, and kitchen staff, most of whom ignored me the remainder of that afternoon's menu review and tasting session. Nice to meet you, too. For the next thirty minutes, Cameron orally deconstructed each culinary offering. Jostling servers and kitchen staff speared the food off each steaming plate. Each item had its own little story, which required me to store and recall scores of menu items, ingredient and process descriptions, appropriate wine pairings, and desserts and aperitifs to recommend. I took a lot of notes.

Tableside preparation techniques required mastery *prior* to performance (a confectioner's torch is as effective at igniting the tablecloth or a diner's chemically infused evening hairstyle as caramelizing the sugar on a crème brûlée). I had to be able to pronounce the Italian and French words on the menu or risk becoming a laughingstock (*amuse-bouche* does not rhyme with *a moose couch)* or worse, gross out the diners (broccoli *rabe* does not rhyme with *rabies*). I had to be Joey Tomatoes.

Cameron then prepared before my eyes one of Zingari's signature dishes: homemade rigatoni pasta *al dente* with cream sauce, peas, sausage, and shavings of Parmesan cheese. He gave me a taste right out of the pan. The pasta was perfect, taut, and it tumbled into my mouth. Cream sauce was the first ingredient that hit my taste buds, encouraging me to chew slowly and enjoy the moment. I soon learned that cooking hand-rolled pasta is an art of its own, and every possible additive of olive oil, sauce, salt, spice, and cheese needed to be precise or it just didn't work. Simple as beauty.

Cameron asked me, "What do you feel after tasting this dish?"

"Joy," I replied, stuffing another helping into my big mouth.

"Yes. An experience. Everything we work toward is helping the customer reach that moment. It's why they come back."

I believe I learned more about food in that moment that at any other during my life, prior or since. As the dinner opening approached, an unspoken sense of urgency began to electrify the air. Everyone scattered to their positions: the servers reviewed scores of choreographed menu sonnets and checked their appearances while the kitchen staff fortified the trenches of each heat delivery station and refrigeration unit prior to that evening's mass assault. I could feel my dead weight. Cameron handed me a binder full of the foundational information necessary for success in my job duties. The most important chapters were dedicated to upselling the customer, the art of encouraging diners to wash down superfluous desserts with egregiously marked-up wines and spirits selling for one-tenth of the price at the liquor store across the street, adding rising yeast to the bill and larger gratuity base. If a server upsold $150, the restaurant took in the additional income with very little overhead while the server saw his gratuity increased by $37.50. A nice return for nominal effort. The Joey Special.

Cameron told me to come back on Saturday night to follow around a master server. "You're going to shadow Lorenzo. Watch everything he does!" The shadow was the restaurant industry's equivalent of a student driver, acting first as the master server's nodding, silent, and smiling toady before graduating to the lackey role of delivering mangled descriptions of evening specials and wine pairings to uncomfortable diners as the master server looked on aghast. Entitled to minimum wage and no share of the tips, the shadowing apprentice over a week's training acquired the basic skill sets or found other work. Swam or drowned. I went home and began to study.

I arrived early the next afternoon and introduced myself to Lorenzo. He looked in his fifties or sixties, with a prominent nose, a disproportionately large, bald, oblong head, shag-carpeted eyebrows, and bright, bathroom-tile teeth. Raised somewhere in southern Italy. Decades of restaurant experience. His expression of disappointment and betrayal in discovering my unmerited inclusion on the weekend schedule was remarkably similar to Cameron's. He explained that my fellow servers had had to prove themselves during the less hectic and less lucrative breakfast, lunch, and early weekday dinner shifts before graduating to the Thursday-through-Sunday prime-time lineup where the big money was earned. Joey Poseur's spot on the roster was not earned and everyone knew it.

Lorenzo was a professional server. His Zen demeanor and radiant smile tempted harried, hungry guests to let down their guard and enjoy the moment. With impeccable posture and language, he was able to describe every appetizer, entrée, side dish, and dessert on Zingari's menu. Lorenzo's ability to upsell—"I wanted to let you know that we have one last 2002 Jordan Cabernet Sauvignon Alexander Valley in the cellar to pair with your filet mignon . . . for $178"—made him a favorite with management. It all came down to money. Zingari's restaurant bar and tabletop space meter ran at a rate of approximately $100 to $150 per hour after factoring in $15 appetizers, $20 glasses of wine, $35 entrees, a 7.5 percent sales tax, and a 20 percent gratuity. In the restaurant industry, the fantasy always came first, with the bill holding off its appearance until it was all over. The check's arrival, like the morning sun, awakened the aggrieved cheapskates, who entered whiny pleas for billing waivers—"Hey, I only drank water" or "I don't remember eating that!"—as well as the mathematicians, who whipped out reading glasses and calculators to compute their undervalued shares by allocating all taxes and gratuities to the remainder of the table. But legally, the customer wasn't right anymore.

I shadowed Lorenzo for the remainder of the week. Put in long hours. Made a lot of mistakes and issued a lot of apologies, but from this sustained effort acquired like gold coins the skills necessary to manage my own section. Lorenzo even shared his tips with me on my last night of training. Logistics under control, I put my sales background to work, quickly becoming a leading upseller. "Jack, Beverly did not get all dressed up to choke down Sutter Home white zinfandel with dinner. Let me show you a nice pinot noir from the Sonoma Valley for $120." Matanzas Creek Joey. Joey Grapes. It took me about a month to feel like I was contributing. The reward was an invitation to hang out with the crew after closing, a man among men and women. We pounded beers and cocktails, enjoyed some of the best food I've ever eaten in my life, and often ended up at someone's apartment to smoke cigarettes and weed. More drinking and mutual affection. I got to hang with people who loved food, wine, music, and late nights— who lived life *every* night.

# Chapter 16

## Joey Rebound
### (1998)

Mind, body, and spirit restored by healthy eating, spiritual study, meditation, psychotherapy, rock climbing, weightlifting, and friends and family, I felt fully charged, heart pumping thunder and lightning. Whatever it was lifted. The brightness of my monitor turned up. My skies were blue again. I heard birds. The thawing crackle of a wintered season. Optimism. Curiosity. Anticipation. Due to rock climbing and healthy eating, I had dropped twenty-five pounds of flab and put on fifteen pounds of muscle, thinning my face and profile. My temporary leave of absence from living made my heart grow fonder of every life, particularly my own. While I continue to suffer brief bouts of despair and panic to this day, the disease has not played a leading role in my life. Joey Survivor. Still Kicking Joey.

To find work in my industry, I went with what had gotten me there and thought about my former colleagues until I recalled and contacted my friend Wayne Weber, a fellow sales executive and top producer from Merrill's Los Angeles office. Wayne was now with Bowne & Co. on the financial printing side of the document management services division. A few days later, Wayne talked to Jo Jacobson, a senior vice president and corporate rock star in the San Francisco office of Bowne. About a week later I received a call from Nick Kane, the executive vice president of Bowne & Co., asking me to lunch at Le Central in Union Square the next day.

Bowne & Co., founded in 1775, is the second oldest company in the country and the oldest publicly traded corporation in the United States, with offices and affiliates worldwide. In 1995, four years prior to my interview, Bowne grossed more than $500 million in revenue. In 1997, more than $700 million—a 40 percent increase. By 1999, nearly $1 billion. I happened to be in the right place at the right time. Sort of. Advancements in digital technology cut tree-pulping demand for ink and paper printing, for scans, copies, and storage. While Bowne survives to this day, the company's revenue declined during the first decades of the new millennium, and it was eventually acquired by R. R. Donnelley in 2010 for only $400 million. But at the time I was interviewing, seismic events altering the culture, economy, and industries of the nation were still eight hundred days away.

I arrived at the restaurant at exactly noon, informing the maître d' I was there to meet Nick Kane.

"Mr. Kane is seated at his table, sir. Please follow me."

His table?

As we approached Nick's table, the maître d' announced, "Mr. Kane, the ex-copy salesman turned failed entrepreneur currently waiting tables a few blocks away has arrived." Okay, maybe not in those words. Nick appeared to be in his early sixties, with archetypal cotton-boll hair from worrying and a bulbous black-cherry nose from too many cocktail parties. I felt comfortable immediately, like I was hanging out with my grandfather. My illusory lemonade-and-porch swing scene instantly disintegrated when Grandpa hurled a knuckleball down the throat of the interview strike zone.

"So, Joseph, tell me about yourself— something I could not learn from your resume."

So much for foreplay. My soul decided to swing for the fences.

"I wasn't prepared," I blurted out. "And every failure I have ever experienced in my life is directly traceable to my own laziness. I didn't do my homework, sir, and I paid the price. I thought I could sell something without historical knowledge of the industry, or without having the necessary respect of those that do. My latest failure was all mine, Nick." I heard the crack of the bat in my mind.

For a long second, Nick did not speak or move. I could not tell if he was touched or disappointed. Then he smiled, his posture warming slightly. "That was a wonderfully honest response, Joseph." Home run. As if on cue, two waiters

placed our meals before us. Cheers. Nick reciprocated by
sharing details of his career challenges. We shared our struggles with anxiety. The exchanges were authentic, the weather
never making an appearance. At precisely 1 p.m., the maître
d' informed Nick that his car had arrived. Nick signed the
check. We stood up and placed our napkin blankets on the
table. Nick tipped the maître d'—"Thank you, Christian"—
and escorted me to the sidewalk, where a shiny black town car
awaited him. Nick turned to me and shook my hand.

"Joseph, it was a pleasure to meet you, and I can say
with confidence that lunch was one of the most enjoyable in-
terviews I have experienced in quite some time. Your candor
is refreshing. While we don't have any openings in financial
sales currently, I'll keep your resume on hand. I really think
you would be a good addition to our team someday."

Free lunch *and* a compliment. I cannot recall how I
replied. I may have just stood there grinning stupidly as his
car drove away. Bitter that he had no openings, but sweet that
he wanted me on the team.

Someday arrived quickly. Two days later, I received a
call from Nick inviting me to fly to LA to meet members of
Bowne's executive team. Twenty-two hours later, I was sitting on a plane next to Nick, reviewing the roster of sales
executives. I took notes like Cliff. Bowne's production facility
was the largest of its kind in the world. We pulled into the
plant and greeted the reception and security personnel. I received an authorization badge. Playing hanger-on to one of
Bowne's executive vice presidents was good for my self-
esteem. I was *somebody*. I could have been a mathematical

genius from RAND ("Thank you for coming, Dr. Dumont") brought in to decipher some elusive code sequence necessary to access a tranche of encrypted data. Or Agent Dumont from the US Securities and Exchange Commission making a surprise regulatory compliance visit. Or Joey Stark.

Installed in each well-appointed executive office was a large window overlooking a factory floor massive enough to house the Millennium Falcon and the remainder of the rebel alliance, refracting the light of two alien worlds through double-paned glass, each essential and accountable to the other. Size mattered in the printing industry. Eliciting memories of the surreal contraptions illustrated by Dr. Seuss, the twenty-five-foot Heidelberg presses resembled train car couplings, requiring ladders and stairs and platforms for the pressman to access, operate, and maintain the thousands of switches, buttons, gears, cogs, panels, and circuits controlling scores of skull-crushing industrial steel rollers. Colossal scrolls of paper like fallen pillars of a biblical temple. Merrill was David to Bowne's Goliath.

For the next five hours, I discussed my ridiculous resume, spilling my sack of beans in front of every wide-eyed manager and vice president, orating the peaks and valleys of my ten-year Homeric odyssey—my treks through the consuming sands of denial and floating-turd swamps of greed, fraud, and betrayal, my battles with a Cyclops ego, my chemical toilet of a father, my existential and financial struggles, scars, and epiphanies—while keeping on the down-low my recent foray into the food service industry. Didn't want to provide too much information. On the way back to the airport, Nick

asked me if I was available to meet Paul David at a gala
Bowne was hosting at the Legion of Honor in San Francisco
in a few weeks. I told him I could move some things around. I
ran home to tell everyone everything in multiple installments
and parallel versions over the next few days. I called Mom.

I heard from Nick about a week later. After providing
the details of the Bowne Gala, he invited me to a Stanford
baseball home game. Told me to bring a date. On Saturday, I
drove to Palo Alto and fell in line with the other vehicles
creeping into the parking facilities surrounding the Stanford
athletic fields. The Bowne event resembled the Dawn at the
Downs Breakfast Gala at the Kentucky Derby, domed by a
white canopy large enough to accommodate a small circus,
with "Bowne & Co." printed in large, dark letters on a gleaming white banner. Beautiful, smiling Bowne emissaries
approached and guided us into the photosphere. Trays of glass
menagerie spirits. I gulped down a vodka cranberry and took a
look around, spotting Nick and his wife chatting with two
other couples, all attired in layers of Stanford regalia. "Uh
oh," I thought, "Someone is going to ask me where I went to
college." My mind began running ten-second trailers, each
hypothetical outing my lack of academic credentials for public
ridicule like a pair of peed pants. My ego's proposed strategies included denial ("Maybe the topic of formal education
won't ever come up at a university event); creativity ("You
never heard of Pikes Peak Junior Technical University in
Rhode Island? Great liberal arts curriculum!"); self-
deprecation ("Just to clarify, I dropped out of junior college");

even cognitive dissonance ("The better question is where did I NOT go to college!").

Fortunately, custom and common courtesy required me to showcase my date who just happened to be incredibly vibrant, adorable, and charming—a match for anyone twice her age. Within minutes, she and the rest of the circle were laughing and exhibiting the body language of old friends. Sometimes it isn't who you are, but the person with whom you arrive. Then Nick called over an impressively built, fashionably dressed man and his pretty wife to join our circle. "Spencer, we're considering Joseph for a sales spot in our San Francisco office. Joseph, please meet Spencer and his wife, Caroline. We were lucky enough to hire Spencer recently for our Palo Alto office. He used to play football for Stanford." I didn't like where this was going. Spencer, however, deflected the softball of an opportunity to make himself the center of the group's admiration. "To be clear," he said, "they only let me on the field if we were leading by more than thirty points." A masterful disarming use of the phrase *let me*. I suspected Spencer had just connected with anyone who had ever warmed a bench. My ego was impressed. Take the compliment *without* being a dick. Apparently, you can learn a lot at Stanford.

The conversations continued to spark as we made our way to our reserved section and settled in to enjoy the game. In the third inning, I heard the smack of aluminum and hard rubber followed by gasps and shouts from surrounding spectators, my peripheral vision glimpsing a fast-approaching, topspinning projectile rising and arching over the first base

line toward our group. Keeping sight of the ball, I stabilized
my stance, extended my right arm like Scotty Smalls, and
reached out barehanded. I heard a skin-on-skin slap. Felt searing heat as the ball spot-welded to my palm. A half note of
silence as the audience confirmed whether to cheer (ball safe-
ly caught), groan (ball dropped), or gasp (ball knocked
someone unconscious). The crowd roared. On some level, I
did not make the catch—we all did. Nick reacted as if I had
just won the World Series, his entire body trembling, the con-
tents of his drink splashing on the sleeves of his Stanford
sweater, a look of ecstasy on his ruddy face. I handed Nick the
ball.

"That was spectacular, Joseph!" he said. "Did you
play ball in college?"

Learning from Spencer's example, I deflected. "No,
sir. Just a lucky catch." Any one of you could have done the
same thing. High fives and back slaps.

***

Two weeks later, it was time to meet Paul David. The Legion
of Honor Museum in San Francisco's Golden Gate Park is an
architectural facsimile of the French Pavilion at the 1915 Pan-
ama Pacific International Exposition. It overlooks Lincoln
Park, with flanking views of the Golden Gate Bridge in the
distance and lily pads in contrasting shades of Crayola green
on the public golf course below. This institution regularly
houses and exhibits rare and valuable archeological artifacts.
Basking in the surreal sights and sounds of success, my mind

wandered and stumbled across an admonishing superego: *Excuse me, young man. This party is for guests. Grab a tray and get to work, asshole!* My date asked me why I had winced. I requested, promptly received, and downed two flutes of effervescent Napa Valley bubbly from a server who looked just like me.

Nick was easy to spot, holding court in a semicircle populated with many of the gang from the Stanford game. I was greeted like a returning soldier. Nick retold the story of "the Catch." Like a war story. The genuine camaraderie stitched on the baseball field cloaked me in a flag of confidence as I strutted around the track in Bowne's home stadium. Connecting at the most basic level with the people with whom you want to build a professional career is the sweet spot of my God-given skills. I've always been able to bond with the pack, and to initiate courageous and confident conversations, some of which now involved catching a foul ball. For that moment, I felt like I belonged.

Paul David, tall and straight, attired in black, with a military bearing and dark-molded Fisher-Price-person hair, presented as someone not to be disturbed. Definitely the wrong candidate for the full Joey. Paul looked tired. We talked only briefly before he patted me on the back. "Let's go have fun with our colleagues." Colleagues? *What just happened? Did I get the job?*

Nick called the next day and told me Bowne was sending me a formal offer. I am sure I said something appropriate in response. After my brief stint in the big leagues with Merrill, and my time spent back in the grapefruit league, I had just been acquired by a billion-dollar company and guaranteed a starting position. I was a player again. I hung up and barfed in the sink. Congratulated myself in the mirror. Ran around the apartment. Barbaric yawps. Landing a dream job is the heroin of masculinity, the metastasizing gamma radiation enhancement of muscularity, performance, and aggression. Hulk Joey. The Bowne's financial gift basket represented new personal best mile markers in base salary, commissions, and bonus potential, a robust expense account and car allowance, a bigger penis, brass balls, a chip on each shoulder. No need to haggle. I accepted the offer. Scheduled an HR appointment. Nick asked his team to gather: "Everyone, I would like to introduce you to the newest member of our executive sales team, formerly of Merrill Corporation, Joseph Dumont!"

## Chapter 17

---

## Joey Revenge of the Douchebags
(1998-2001)

The entire Bowne executive sales team met every Monday morning at 8:30 a.m. in a cafeteria-sized conference room dominated by a fallen tree of a conference table surrounded by two dozen high-backed black leather chairs, nameless and interchangeable. Sales began at sunrise. The early bird gets to keep his job. In American business, Monday represents the prime-time slot of every sales manager's weekly goals. Plans are reviewed. Reports summarized. Financial pipeline assessed. Compliments. Pro forma revenue discussions. Leads. Reminders of quarterly performance metrics. Success markers for the week. Daily objectives. A reminder to be careful out there. At this level, it was not enough to hit the ground running, whatever that means. Instead, a well-compensated sales executive's revenue figures were expected to take off and soar to new heights with quicker departure times. In these zero-sum games, those unable to fly were dive-bombed and devoured by those able to rise. We are all scared of being eaten.

Bowne had installed as my team's quarterback Jo Jacobson, the company's top sales revenue producer whose integrity, skill sets, and accomplishments likely would have propelled her to success at any endeavor at any time in history. She was my hero. I met Jo through my tenure at Merrill, where she was also a top performer. When Jo retired, she held some of the highest statistical sales records in Bowne and Co.'s two-hundred-and-twenty-year history.

It's better at the top. Much better. The focus of my first Bowne executive sales meeting was the upcoming US Open Golf Championship hosted at the Olympic Club in San Francisco. Founded in 1860 and operating to this day, the Olympic Club is the oldest private country club in our nation, its guarded perimeter containing not one, not two, but three world-class golf courses. Because three is better than two. As they had at the Stanford baseball game, Bowne walled off its own Vatican City with bottle service and pretty servers, creating for its distinguished guests a more exclusive space from which to observe others and be seen doing so. Even better, I was not expected to carry anyone's bag, measure an inside leg, or refire a still-squirming steak.

Every client wanted a golden ticket to tour the WASP Fun Factory: puffy white marshmallow tent, catered gastronomical novelties, legions of fizzy-lifting drinks, wine cellar, berries, cream, bubbles, music, and a chocolate river (okay, maybe not a chocolate river). Coverage of the exclusive event and its distinguished invitees would be beamed to the rest of the world by satellite. A target-rich environment in which to engage with investment bankers, venture capitalists, corporate counsel, scientists, software engineers, and any person knighted with an acronym of corporate success: CEO, CFO, CTO, CMO, COO, ESQ. Anyone connected to a startup filing an imminent IPO.

My new industry was about to be disrupted by all things digital. My grandfather's seemingly eccentric alliterative axiom, "Church, computers, cars, in that order," with computers positioned between God and commerce, the metaphysical and material, felt prescient. Even conservative, federally regulated financial institutions such as banking, insurance, and the stock market sought to take advantage of new technologies to reach formerly untapped customer populations. Digital media warped time and space by decreasing transactional time integrals from minutes to seconds to fractions of seconds in multiple discourse mediums and communities, including interpersonal, commercial, and scientific, shaping American culture in its own image: digital information, digital economies, digital media, digital discovery, digital security, digital plus noun; the list was infinite.

This renaissance of media technologies developed radical interactive technologies that reformed commercial markets and logistics: new modes of finance, advertising, and customer service; the enhanced ability to track supply chains, delivery, and return information; advances in digital records technology and increased storage capacity; even reformed operational and executive structures of involved business entities. Virgin markets in interactive commerce technology attracted pioneers seeking to prospect veins of intellectual property, develop new thoughts, words, codes, devices, mine data oceans and opportunities, and monetize these newly discovered concepts into IPOs. Netscape's web browser technology provided customers with exponential access to the burgeoning connectivity and commercial potential of the internet. Google's search engine technology made the internet easy to use. Amazon would become synonymous with e-commerce, beginning with books and evolving into the corporate monster that dominates the industry today. TiVo would forever change our television experience with a DVR technology that allowed digitized video on hard disk for data storage, quickly replacing the VCR and its blinking red clock. And PalmPilot would introduce the first handheld PDA, the precursor to the smartphones now ubiquitous in our purses and pockets. Everything was changing. And not all of it was good. But at the time, it never occurred to me that we were all trapped in a bubble. Or that bubbles float only because they hold nothing inside.

The same technological developments blowing oxygen into the raging bonfire of the stock market would over the next decade burn down entire production divisions in the printing industry by suffocating commercial demand for ink and paper services, deforesting the business model of Bowne, its competitors, and my profession. I developed a friendship with a young lawyer named Greg—midthirties, an expert in federal regulations governing venture financing and IPOs. Over drinks we discussed tech-industry news, stock prices and trends, personal contacts within the industry, and talked about motorcycles. And one day during a long lunch, he just blurted out, "You're in no immediate danger of losing your job, Joseph, but Bowne will not be around in ten years." And then he took another bite of his sandwich.

The printing industry was only one of many casualties of digital technology. Previously viable businesses based on the group's dependence on a select individual's access to necessary, timely, and accurate information would be altered, displaced, or destroyed: small retail shops dependent on continuous neighborhood foot traffic; businesses unable to compete with a larger competitor's superior resources, economies of scale, and ability to implement new technology into their existing business model; businesses whose monopolies on information were busted by free public access to the world's information through the Promethean internet.

Prior to these systemic changes, Bowne's inability to bridge the generational chasm between its aptly named senior sales staff and a start-up's scientists and executives who were often only a decade out of high school was costing the company a fortune in lost revenue. Nick hired thirty-two-year-old Joey Cool to talk to the popular kids about landing these IPO accounts, a part similar to the influencer role I played in high school—nurturing new relationships with scores of classmates on campus, athletic competitions, and illegal parties, linking friends with other friends in the pre-Facebook era. I supplemented my personal outreach tactics by reading technology industry publications such as *Red Herring Magazine*, *Fast Company*, *InfoWorld*, *The Industry Standard*, and *The Recorder*, and newly published websites such as Hotwired and

Yahoo, and blogs and chat rooms no longer living, where technology and business news overflowed the banks of networks and platforms at electric light speeds.

It was my job to get to know these new pioneers and the rich men that financed them, connecting through as many mediums as possible: in person, over the phone, in writing. To get my number on their speed dial, my smiling picture on their credenza at work in matching golf shirts, and to be invited to a family BBQ at their beach house—which was integral to secure seven-figure contracts with multiple signatories and affixed notary affidavits—and then to nurture indefinitely these newly minted relationships until they graduated into friendships. We work with those we like.

Reformed by Bowne's faith, hope, charity, and large paycheck, I quickly scrapped the many humble lessons discovered through my pursuit of Eastern philosophy, the practices focused on spirit and mindfulness. I reprised enthusiastically the role of Joey Storm, King of the Dipshits. It was time to make some money!

I'd been chasing for some time Frank Siskowski, the CFO of E-Loan, who was directing an exciting company toward an impending IPO. Sporting a custom gray three-button suit, stick pin, and fat watch—the dress uniform of the corporate elite guard—I drove over to E-Loan's Dublin, California, headquarters to hand deliver to him Bowne's carefully crafted proposal to handle E-Loan's IPO filing. Frank met me in the lobby wearing a slightly rumpled button-down shirt and khakis. He looked me over and said with a wry smile, "If you want my deal, Joseph, you can't come in here lookin' like that."

The office was a big open space with numerous dry-erase whiteboards marked with Venn diagrams and conceptual models, Cartesian grids of bars and graphs, and the names of evolving concepts of computer science and media technology. There was the obligatory ping-pong table, empty cheese-stained pizza boxes, old cans of Red Bull and Mountain Dew, empty paper cups, coffee machine, and men: young men, men in short pants and flip-flops, men in jerseys and sneakers, all planted in rows between keyboards and NASA-inspired private monitors, staring affectionately at rapidly appearing light-bright lines of code generated by the electricity of their thoughts and busy fingers. One young coder asked me if I was a congressman.

I began to keep jeans, T-shirts, and retro tennis shoes in the back of my truck for quick wardrobe changes in parking lots outside the buildings of my IPO appointments. And with increased frequency, I would ride my motorcycle to appointments and enter the meetings with helmet in hand. I got to know these young leaders as people. I listened. I read recommended readings. I sat and thought, trying to put it all together. If tech commerce represented the missing link in the economic evolution of the world, then I would learn its codes and speak the dialects of its language and attempt to surf the very same tidal wave about to land on my career in the printing industry. I landed the E-Loan IPO. Nick was elated. It was a high-profile and high-valued transaction that provided

Bowne & Co. with a seven-figure payday. I was on top of the world again and looking forward to the next deal.

***

The coin of an unlimited expense account has two sides. Heads depicts the array of props made available to the salesman to cast his illusions to the customer for his specific consumption, entertainment, and enjoyment of an audience suspended in disbelief. Tails, however, represents the requirement that an unlimited expense account be linked to an unlimited credit line. The executive sales professionals at Bowne, pampered with six-figure salaries, fat bonuses, and commissions, were justifiably expected to use their own credit lines to carry business expenses until the company's next reimbursement period. This was a potential career-ending problem for me, reminding me that past failures can haunt a man's game for years to come, no matter how much forward momentum he has. No banking institution, even those willing to gamble in roulette-wheel probabilities wanted anything to do with a recently evicted delinquent debtor with no net worth and an arctic credit rating. Teams of debt collectors hunted me like I was Bin Laden.

Time to call Mom. Mom had overcome her own gauntlet of financial challenges since Dad had left her alone in 1974 with a blank credit history. Mom's credit was good because she posed no risk. At first, she could not understand why I needed to become an additional signatory on one of her credit card accounts: "Why doesn't this Bowne issue you a credit card? You should be able to pay the bill with all that good money you're making. Why aren't all those big, fancy businesspeople paying for their own suppers? Your Grandpa Probert never used a credit card." All valid points. Mom would have been dangerous with a law license. But she agreed in writing to cover and carry my flotilla of business expenses, unconditionally.

Nonetheless, my palms were sweaty when I slipped my gleaming new credit card into the chocolate-colored leather folder containing a torn-off slip of skinny paper requesting immediate payment of over $2,000 for an opulent dinner to which I had treated the executive team of Next Level Technology in one of Manhattan's finest restaurants. I resisted the urge to grab the waiter's wrist when he picked up the folder and slow-walked it back to the verification and processing machine housed in the service station. As I waited for my card to be run and more importantly approved, my mind danced a caffeinated leprechaun jig: *I am sorry, sir. Your mommy's credit card has been declined. She is on the line and wants to speak with you. Perhaps you should consider killing yourself.*

In real life, the folder was brought back gushing the pride of my approval. "Thank you, sir." I signed the merchant slip like a big hero. Then we dashed out into the living streets of New York City and partied like Japanese businessmen: private entrances, pounding music, bottle service, fancy cigars, proximity to pretty, uninhibited young women, Joey's bawdy stories and back-slapping punchlines. I won the Next Level Technology IPO. Thanks, Mom!

Over lunch with my lawyer buddy, Greg, he asked me
if I was interested in being a member of the Olympic Club,
the venerable organization that hosted the US Open during the
first few months of my tenure at Bowne. Greg explained the
club was seeking younger members, men under the age of
thirty-four specifically, to play on the tennis team. He, too,
was a tennis player.

He invited me to the stately six-story brown-brick
Olympic Club manor house located a few blocks from Union
Square. Small placards reading "Private Property" and
"Members Only" conveyed reminders to the literate that the
uninvited were illegal. Tall, white columns flanked quarter-
ton doors. Drawbridge checkpoint. Uniformed sentries monitored incoming members, guests, staff, and service calls. One
validated Greg's membership with a smile. Greg was confirmed. Hanger-on Joey was tolerated. Free to roam.

Plush carpets and custom-woven rugs cushioned the
hand-stitched shoes of patrons attired in blue blazers fastened
with gold-plated buttons and bright-white shirts set off by
fruit-striped neckties. The interior decor was a showcase of
artisans and artists. Ornate stonework. Pillars encased in white
marble. Sturdy walls and tall ceilings constructed with great
ship-worthy beams and planks. Master-crafted staircases and
fireplaces, comforting elevators, countless pieces of wood and
leather library furniture trimmed in gold. Glowing filaments
and countless fixtures of crystal and brass, table-sized por-
traits of ash-and-dust members, trophy cases, trophy shelves,
trophies of all shapes and sizes, banners and medals, sports
regalia and memorabilia, victorious spoils, all a crescendo to

the club's hundred-foot natatorium, an indoor, Olympic-sized swimming pool framed with Doric columns. The ideal set for cinematic depictions of the existential denial and debauchery accelerating the Roman Empire's decline. Like Brookline, I wasn't allowed in this clubhouse either.

The restrooms were staffed with uniformed attendants unable to dissemble micro-expressions of existential agony as they valiantly performed their service duties for men who ignored them. I caught a glimpse of my own guilt in the long, polished mirror as the man at the far end of the long wooden bank of gold-plated sinks and faucets began fiddling with his tiny retinue of colognes, perfumes, breath sprays, tissues, and mints. Something wrong with the whole setup. Two strangers paid to awkwardly share the intimacy of one man's bodily functions until the culminating ceremonial exchange of a clean, white towel. Tip jars and reciprocal nods. I knew right then that I couldn't handle being a member. The club was simply too much for me—or I was not enough for the club. Couldn't put my finger on it.

# Chapter 18

## Joey Interaction
### (2000–2003)

Big job. Amazing girlfriend. Dozens of friends and admirers. Relationships with some of the most powerful people in the Bay Area. Cozy apartment in gold rush San Francisco. Tailored pretty-boy clothing. Jewelry like Mrs. Howell. Gas in the tank. Rolls of cash. Lines of credit and respect. Upgraded status, mileage, and points. Life fast-forwarded. My future began to dream. Joey America the Beautiful. Purple Mountain Joey Majesty.

The demand for commercial media talent created prime opportunities for new species of industry professionals, most under the age of thirty, including the following: (1) programmers who wrote the code, comprising the nerds courted from Stanford, MIT, Caltech, and Carnegie Mellon and lavished with ransom-sized compensation packages; (2) start-up executives charged with scaling the distribution and profitability of the programmers' work product who debated "eye-balls," "traction," "user metrics data," and "algorithms"; (3) technology supply chain and service partners seeking to participate in new markets through new mediums; and (4) professional agents and matchmakers who brought everyone together, who acted as relational translators fluent in technology, business, and human discourse, and who were trusted to answer the question. ? What's in it for me? This was a job for Joey Smooth. I found myself in the enviable position of being well paid to sell financial printing services to hot new companies desperate to hire people able to speak the lucrative language of tech commerce. I fielded streams of insider information and employment offers from start-ups for executive-level sales positions with glamorous titles like "director" and "vice president" that promised six-figure salaries and most importantly foundation-level stock options with potential exponential increases in value. The views from the top of the mountain were breathtaking.

Over dinner at the Birdsalls' one evening, I blathered on about these revelations like a wild-haired prophet, preaching to the owners of a web development agency how new technologies were reshaping the world of commerce. "Oh thanks, Joe," Mo dryly remarked as she plopped more mashed potatoes on my plate, giving me a look usually reserved for Mike. "We had no idea. Tell us more." My face flushed. Mike interjected, "Joe, if you want to be part of real change, you could join our agency and sell our services." Food for thought. That night as I stared at the ceiling, I reflected on the Birdsalls' incredible offer, weighing the risks of entangling the warmth of our personal relationship with the cooler jet streams of sales contacts, service contracts, and bottom-line revenue figures. The tiebreaker was my belief that I would do a good job. The next day, I drove to Birdsall Interactive (BI) to sell myself on a position that had already been offered to me by its owners over buttered spuds. After only a few hours of amicable discussion, I became their vice president of sales.

With his telephone headset, Mike resembled an offensive coordinator of a college football team as he methodically cold-called a hundred companies per day attempting to sell BI's services to marketing departments, just like he had at Print and Copy Factory. Just like I had at Stuart James. But I was a one-on-one sales guy. A camouflaged big game hunter or sniper able to focus intently and patiently on a single target. I would act as wide receiver, contributing with long yardage plays, while Mike would continue grinding out short yardage through dozens of carries. A balanced offense. Smaller in stature yet far more intimidating than her husband, Mo acted as the firm's creative genius, oracle, and existential center of gravity, leading and managing five highly intelligent and talented creative professionals. Mo could have scaled her agency and ruled the world of online advertising if commercial and professional success amounted to her endgame. Mo preferred balance. The agency was an RV to transport the family through life's terrain of basic needs that she and Mike could park in the driveway every night in time for dinner, as opposed to an entity to be monetized and sold one day to the highest bidder. Like I would have done.

Brady Brook was the lead designer. Six foot two with a dense, muscular physique. His brain burned like a lighthouse beacon. Admired by men and women alike, Brady's personality acted as an electromagnet, drawing others into the party of his life. Bob, a gifted artist and musician, went by his last name, Tait, and looked like he commuted up on a wave from Los Angeles, sporting wrinkled T-shirts and shorts and bottle-opening flip-flops. Ian Gilles served as BI's Flash developer—a rare skill set at the time. Wicked smart. Everything infuriated Ian.

Our head of tech was Rob Fife. Six foot four, two hundred and eighty pounds, heavy metal concert T-shirts and long shorts. A man covered in hair, with trunks for legs, big flip-flop feet, and possibly some Wookiee or Sasquatch ancestry, who endured my daily technical inquiries: "What does *http* stand for? What is a server, raid array, or a thin client? Is a floppy disk part of the hard drive?"

David Ford was BI's redheaded executive producer, our Seinfeldian maestro. We were the cool kids surfing the intimidating tidal wave of the internet economy, the hilarious cast of a hip IT sitcom, our own constellation of stars. Untapped talent appeared in unexpected places, including the local Round Table Pizza, where we became acquainted with a young cashier whose name was Robert. Much to our delight and immaturity, Robert disclosed the underutilized developer skills he had mastered over years of deconstructing pornography code. We hired him a week later.

The multibillion-dollar pornography industry accounts for a third of our national internet activity, funded by

billions of rhythmic clicks from millions of pud-tuggers sub-
stituting screen time for the reciprocal warmth of human
relationships. Seems ironic that advancements in digital
transmission speed that innovated surgical procedures, space
exploration, and credit card encryption technologies can be
traced back to the rush to monetize masturbation. Two sides
of the same slippery coin. The internet generated infinite
waves of electronic pornographic images, granting free admission to anyone who was able to get their hands on a
computer. The phrase *surfing porn* made its debut. The industry could now reach out and diddle someone in the comfort
and relative privacy of the family residence without the sticky
access, privacy, and payment concerns related to magazines
and videocassette tapes. Husbands were caught not wearing
the family pants by their disappointed wives, hypnotized by
slow-loading digital porn, mouse in each hand. Nobody gave
much thought to where all this data was going and where it
might lie in wait. Fossilized pecker tracks and deviant browser
histories became subject to judicial review by grossed-out
employers and publication by bad breakuppers. Everything
old was new again. Bet no one saw that coming.

During my time at Bowne and first years at BI, America continued to be the only superpower in the world and was
not involved in any wars. The economy swaggered and business was good. Plenty of six-figure service contracts with
well-known, reputable companies in the Bay Area. BI double-
doubled gross revenue over the next two years, which increased the size of our team, and my responsibilities
proportionately. We even hired someone to count our money.

I paid off my Range Rover, sold it to a retired cable car driver, and put the proceeds down on one of the first Audi TT models available in the United States—a sculpted piece of sophisticated engineering worthy of a James Bond adventure, every shift a hit of ecstasy. I ordered my silver two-seater without a test drive and updated and tweaked the software package, increasing the engine's output forty additional horses after paying well over sticker price. I installed a new custom exhaust, too. 'Cause I was worth it.

The douchebag employs overreaching fashion artistry to draw attention to his physical appearance and expertise: the cape of the superhero; the gunfighter's pistols; beetle-black jacket and boots of the motorcycle rider; the pirate's sword. Jack Sparrow, Napoleon, and Charlie Sheen are douchebags. So too was President George W. Bush when he staged a one-mile flight to a waiting aircraft carrier so he could walk the deck in a flight suit cradling a pilot's helmet to announce we had accomplished our mission in Iraq. The ascot, beret, and leather jacket all fit under the umbrella of douchebaggery. After a decade of tolerating frumpy, conservative dress code policies in the workplace, I created my own rock-star-biker thing: peacock hair, rose-colored aviator shades, dark leather jacket, leather belts with tarantula buckles and wallet chains, precious rocks and magic rings, thick metal watches and bracelets. All of it celebrated the next level of Joey.

The card-house collapse of the first internet economy was yet another manic period in America fueled by illusion, greed, and an intentional suspension of skepticism, a dynamic similar to the speculation bubble that burst in the sixteenth century when a group of European merchants engaged in a futures feeding frenzy over a diseased tulip. So too the fraternity of Silicon Valley capitalists, investors, executives, brokers, technicians, attorneys, and money changers who talked only to each other, and believed all of this was real. In both cases, the tulips were virtual. The rise and fall of the wax-winged internet sock puppet Pets.com told the typical story arc of viral do-nothing companies at the turn of the millennium. In the sweaty bounce-house investing rush in early 2000, the Pets.com IPO raised $120 million (almost $500 million today) by promising investors that pet owners would pounce to pay for the privilege of having too many bags of discount dog food and pet amenities delivered to doorsteps. The customers did not bite. And even if they had, the company failed to install the necessary infrastructure to fulfill its promises, such as factoring in the shipping and handling costs related to relocating an eighty-five-pound bag of dog food. By the end of the year, Pets.com had shit and liquidated all over the front yards of Silicon Valley. Within two years, most similarly situated IPOs would wet the beds of investors.

Shareholders of giant grocery and retail corporations at the turn of the millennium had no qualms about eliminating critical staff positions when they invested obscene amounts of capital into "self-directed checkout" technology to replace human cashiers with computer kiosks. A lot of bottom-line-gazing executives believed they had foreseen a paradigm shift similar to how automated teller machines had allowed banks to operate customer service branches with fewer human tellers. Imagine the savings in labor costs by eliminating the labor. To the dismay of the operators and investors, something unexpected and profound occurred once the robot checkout machines were installed and activated. The public hated them. Most Americans refused to use them. There were a lot of pissed-off shoppers. Twenty years later, helpful human cashiers and baggers continue to ring up, sort, and package our retail purchases, and the shunned Easter Island machines are exiled to the end of the service line. Customers continue to demand the trust-inspiring personal assistance they had always enjoyed when inspecting, pricing, and bagging food for the family table: "Did you find everything you were looking for? This carton is leaking. Let me get you another. I can run a price check on that. Need any help with your bags? Have a nice day." The mostly male tech experts had discounted the human variables when applying their industrial analytics and advice to commercial markets. These and many errors of disconnection went viral.

Although they were intrigued with the benefits of the internet economy, most Americans were not yet prepared to trust new degrees of market attenuation and intangibility. They preferred to conduct business with real people in relatively small spaces and invest with stalwart companies such as General Foods, Ford, and IBM, which produced tangible consumer goods for loyal American families out of brick-and-mortar facilities with neighborhood addresses and employed American workers. Ultimately, even the best carnival barkers were unable to supply any demand for a distant, formless nebula of products and services. The economy recoiled in shock and distress. By mid-2001, bad things began to happen to good companies. The telecommunication companies charged with developing the complex hardware systems capable of running commerce platforms—despite acting in good faith to comply with the crush of speculative demand—crashed under the weight of excessive debt loads. Suppliers and other satellite companies were knocked out of their orbits. Critically wounded companies like WorldCom, Adelphia Communications, and Global Crossings were choked out and pillaged by their own leaders. The dot-com landmine detonated a few months later, damaging markets, reputations, portfolios, and segments of the economy. Then September 11, 2001, shook America like a baby.

For the last quarter of 2001 and the first quarter of 2002, as investors stopped writing checks and consumers stopped placing orders, companies dependent on the public's confidence suffered fiscal heart attacks. Businesses like BI flatlined. Not silence—the held breath of fear. Mike and I employed every tool at our disposal to bring in business, called in every favor. But the streams were empty. The herds had galloped or limped away. Although we had landed our largest account when Hitachi of America hired the agency to redesign their entire web enterprise, BI could no longer sustain itself at its present size and overhead. In early 2003, we laid off half our team, including Joey Weak Sales. I felt more liberated than disappointed when I sold my TT to some hip young guy still employed in technology. I only enjoyed expensive cars when I deserved them.

Chapter 19

---

## The Bachelor Party
### (2003)

Unemployed. Downgraded. Downsized. Circumcised. A plug ripped out from the wall by its cord. In a culture that congratulated long hours of hard work and classified sloth as a deadly sin, involuntary unemployment felt cruel and unusual, solitary and confining, lethal even in small doses. Status demoted from preferred to unauthorized. From insider to trespasser. Dumped to the curb, coveting the secret codes and card keys employed by the good morning coffee people pouring warm into office buildings. I necessarily stopped spending money on nonessentials and discovered this consumer cleansing ritual to be surprisingly calming and therapeutic. My spirit continued to learn from my temporary employment challenges, but my ego ached to be back in the active position of protecting and loving, producing and contributing, inspiring and succeeding. To do whatever it was I was supposed to do. To be big again.

For the first time in my life, I qualified for unemployment benefits: $1,500 per month for up to twelve months based on my employment history with Bowne and BI. Enough to cover rent, utilities, and my castration wound each month until I got back to work. Seemed like a windfall at the time, and I was grateful every time the envelope arrived in the mail. Unemployment claims offices are pit stops for hard workers, those only recently out of the race and likely to reenter within the benefits period with the help of a committed crew. Unemployment benefits are not handouts, aid, welfare, dole, "on the county," or any other shit-smeared label intended to denigrate. Rather, California's unemployment compensation system works like any other form of insurance coverage by pooling "premiums," in this case withheld from wages earned within the state to pay inevitable valid claims. One hundred percent of these subsistence payments transfuse immediately back into the local economy when the beneficiary pays forward their monthly rent, food, and healthcare insurance expenses, allowing the capital to continue running downstream. Everybody benefitted. I had legally and ethically earned this compensation. So why did I feel so emasculated about filing a claim?

I walked down to the EDD for the City and County of San Francisco housed on the corner of Turk and Franklin, a nondescript yellow cake-batter building with four layers of blueberry windows, the only adornment on the exterior being a small metal state seal. Feeling small, I tugged open the thick-paned glass door, changing the air pressure and temperature of the room. Some of the other displaced workers looked up or over a shoulder before losing interest. Everyone settled in for a long morning. Not like we had jobs to get to. When thrown into circumstances of misery or embarrassment, most of us take comfort in the company of others similarly situated—the more the merrier—implying a psychological benefit to recognizing there are other people as screwed as you are. For some, it is the beginning of empathy.

I waited in chairs with an array of people: electricians, carpenters, drivers, and machinists of every race for whom the union had no assignments that week, many wearing lumbar braces, broken down by the continuous repetitive physicality required in their industries, hard labor ground into their clothing; restaurant and retail store associates, male and female, decades of work history reliving the same seasons, laid off or no longer able to keep up with better-looking employees half their age; women wearing safe shoes; panicked middle class white guys, some like me from the tech industry, others gray-haired and enfeebled, presenting as aggrieved, wallet lifted; middle-aged women wearing accessories of former status. We checked in with staff and completed intake forms. Authenticated identity with driver's licenses, social security cards, and passports. Waited some more. Stood in line at the window. Eventually completed the application procedures and mandatory filing forms before being patted on the head and excused. By the time I got home, I felt I had worked a full day.

I woke up the next morning feeling invisible. Snoozed until shrilled out of bed by teapot anxiety. Checked messages for huge job offers. Wasted time on the internet. Stood sadly in the shower. Filled the remaining seven hours of everyone else's workday with distractions, new humiliations, and cramps and acid triggered by corrupted ruminations of inner-space exploration. I played a lot of golf. Decreased my PlayStation Tiger Woods golf handicap to subzero tempera-tures and captured a string of major tournament championships by virtue of my four-hundred-yard drives, my GPS short game, and a regimen of performance-enhancing, class-one-felony medical grade marijuana. But video games were not as fun when you had too much time to play them. Finally, it was bedtime: my thoughts adrift for hours on a catastrophizing ocean, my ego clinging to wreckage of my remembered life. Anyway. How was *your* day?

I interviewed at a few mature advertising agencies and one with an infant start-up in Berkeley where my buddy Scotty served as an executive. While every graduate of the Wharton School at the University of Pennsylvania is entitled to highlight the bragging fact of their attendance on a resume, Wharton would likely reference Scotty's years of attendance and degree award on its resume. I earned enough points dur-ing our recently kindled relationship to make the cut for his upcoming bachelor party in Las Vegas. My job hunter called me the following Monday about a small advertising agency specializing in market research and web design founded in 1998 by two men in their early thirties, Jeff Rosenblum and Jordan Berg. They were looking for a head of business devel-opment. I wasn't overly interested, but not wanting to be a dick I called Jeff anyway and left a voicemail. When I didn't hear back after three days, I figured I was out of the running.

On my way to the airport Thursday for a long fraternal weekend, I noticed a voicemail: "Joey fucking Dumont, this is Jeff Rosenblum . . . I'm sitting here in Scotty's limo on our way to Vegas for his bachelor party, and we're going to drink our fuckin' faces off this weekend . . . Can't wait to hang out, dude!" Too clear and cogent for a butt dial. Why was Jeff Rosenblum sending me a message about my friend Scotty's bachelor party instead of offering me a job interview? Then the epiphany. Holy shit. Scotty's Jeff and my job hunter's Jeff were the same person. In a few moments, I would commence my first bachelor party job interview in the sticky, kaleidoscopic briar patch of Las Vegas. I've rarely been happier.

Las Vegas is a douchebag destination spot. Liquor. Lust. Gratuitous nudity. Dark light. Drumming techno music. Black-market pharmaceuticals. Cavernous restaurants and clubs. Vegas is where men go to pretend to be bigger men, better men, to walk the hallways of manufactured castles, temples, and tombs mimicking the sets where once great blood-and-bone men, conquerors, pharaohs, captains, rock stars, crooners, emperors, and kings paraded with lusty entourages. The land of victorious spoils. Luxor. Caesar's Palace. Treasure Island. Excalibur. Steve Wynn's giant ego museum. Joey's Mecca.

Vegas rewards fluency in American Alpha Male Dialect. Trash talk. Bawdy talk. Big money talk. Locker room talk. Dick talk. Guy talk. Overheard in war zones, garages, bars, warehouses, restaurant kitchens, man caves, and trading floors. On docks, construction sites, and every form of media. All you need is a group of guys and some finite resources. More monkeys than bananas. At its shallow surface level, guy talk celebrates the talker's personal conquests related to male membership, status, money, intellect, or potency *relative* to another man's deficiencies under the same criteria. I am awesome *because* you suck. Irony is mandatory. Mocking a man's bed-wetting child with special needs is obviously out of bounds, but implying your hugely successful buddy overcame special-needs challenges during *his* bed-wetting childhood is roast-worthy material. Points are awarded for artistry ("Dude, your teeth are so big they look like stand-up urinals") and tastelessness ("That's not what your mother said last night"). Always helpful to analogize some facet of your friend to other disfavored groups—the iconic "You play ball like a girl," for instance, employs one tightly packed simile to take down another man by denigrating the throwing motion of all women. Like a grenade.

But on a deeper level, the gist of our guy-talk language, bravado, and embellishments serves as the pre-contest linguistic ritual of any pack, squad, or legion. Because a *real man* strives to outlive his daily trials and persistent ego and become something invulnerable to a world without pause. We're supposed to be brave. Rise each day. And the day after that. Be a hero. Be gainfully employed. Be macho. Be strong. Or lose our Man Status.

I found the growing pack of alpha dogs staked out in the blackjack pen of the hotel casino. Quick ceremonies of proud introductions between laureates in Scotty's life. Thursday afternoon cocktail servers bobbing and weaving through a pack of proud males in starched collared shirts and overpriced jeans delivering competing oratories and ballads of epic greatness and brutal failures, all with happy endings. Shots firing in all directions. Hits and stays and busts. Orphaned cash. Throwing-star playing cards. Privileged credit cards lounging on plastic rafts. Moments before the hunt.

When I walked up and hugged Scotty, Jeff heard my name, disengaged from his conversation, and advanced in my direction, fronted by the thumping turbulence of his baritone voice. "Joey fucking Dumont! Shirts-off hugs, dude!" he said, peeling his shirt off as he approached like a gorilla. Since I loved taking off my clothes too, I pulled off my own shirt. We hugged like cavemen on the casino floor until a look from the pit boss implied that further acts of indecency would be met with overwhelming counter action and concrete feet. Everything about Jeff was big. Six foot one and confidently handsome, Jeff was a walking electromagnetic pole with an ion-charged personality who also happened to own two of the largest ears I'd ever seen in my life. Like head-mounted satellite dishes. The size that got caught in doors or made elephants fly. People sometimes asked to touch them. Jeff often referenced his pair of potato chip protuberances in self-effacing conversation starters. Jeff introduced Jordan as his best friend and business partner. Jordan looked like a younger Paul Newman, well-groomed but dressed more for a Cambridge regatta than a Vegas casino: sweater vest, polo shirt, Dockers, Sperry Top-Siders, bold socks. Intelligent and measured, Jordan played Rocky to Jeff's Bullwinkle. Teller to Jeff's Penn. Nobody had any trouble telling them apart.

We stayed in trios in large, well-appointed suites. Preparing for our quiet evening, I'd brought a T-shirt that I'd recently bought in Italy with "WASTED" printed in big, black letters across the chest overlaying an orange-and-black lava lamp pattern. An obnoxious Chrome Hearts belt buckle on a thick, highway-black leather belt crowning disintegrating designer jeans. Two Green Lantern rings on each hand. Unnecessary motorcycle boots. Empty wallet and chain. Cement sun-god spiked hair. Ready to go. After gorging on forty-pound elephant steaks and punctured casks of California wine at an opulent chop-and-slaughter house, our squad marched over to the Ghostbar at the Palms Hotel. Vegas clubs were cashing in on the new reality TV genre by paying "reality stars" to make guest appearances: Johnny Knoxville and his jackasses, Ashton Kutcher and his punks, women named Tequila, unemployable and unrecognizable former child stars searching for one more moment of adoration before the inevitable drug overdose. The entrance line resembled a better-looking airport security screening. Of course, we had no intent of waiting our turn to get in. The Wharton Class of Not Joey already had big jobs with heavy paychecks, earning more in a month than the median annual income for a family of four. Brett, a vice president of international marketing for MTV, explained to the security agent that he represented twenty douchebag executives buzzing in bachelor-party mode who were ready to drop $10,000 into the club's coffers over the next few hours. Less than a minute passed before a mountainous bouncer escorted our group to our small, roped-off private section, one in an archipelago of private islands surrounded by an ocean teeming with schools of frustrated patrons laying siege to the bar and searching for a place to stand.

VIP sections with *bottle service* were created with the American douchebag in mind. Imagine a black-windowed, supersized Denny's or Applebee's with velvet ropes segregating the booths from the counter and commons areas offering two tiers of service for grossly disparate menu prices. Stud farms and pretty-pony sections. The club coerces the ponies in twenty-dollar installments: cover charge; watered-down vodka Red Bulls, martinis, and cosmopolitans; gratuities to overworked servers and bathroom attendants. But clubs go all-out for the stallions, charging $600 for a bottle of premium vodka, $25 for bottles of Bud Lite, $20 for bottles of water, $100 for finger-food platters, all served by shockingly beautiful and scantily clad women, running train lines of unrequested ice buckets and fruit, ("More of everything!"), the aggregate marked up another 25 percent. Fuck you very much. God, I loved this shit.

Just after midnight, Paris Hilton and her gaggle of baby ducklings were escorted by a bouncer into the section next to ours. It might have been the alcohol, or the fact that he aspired to impress the pack with his formidable charisma, but Jay, a major executive at a large tech company in the Valley, imbued with the placid confidence of a serial killer, yelled into my ear, "Joey, I'm going to ask Paris to come over and join us. Will you be my wingman?"

"I would be honored, buddy," I said.

Jay had striking good looks framed by a diurnal five o'clock shadow, but he was also a deal-breaking couple of inches shorter than Paris in her three-inch heels. I was more than happy to act as Jay's black box recording final communications before the crash. We did a shot of tequila. But before we launched the mission, six-foot-five Jeremy Shockey, Pro Bowl tight end for the New York Giants, a two-hundred-sixty-pound Thor-like man, avalanched into our path, intercepting Paris's complete attention. She immediately squealed, "Jeremy!" as she jumped into his arms and wrapped her legs around him. I leaned over and shouted to Jay.

"Dude, you're not going to take that. Kick his ass!" Everyone laughed. Jay took it like a man.

# Chapter 20

## Joey Big Apples
### (2003)

Monday morning my phone rang. It was Jeff.

"Dude, can we reschedule our interview for sometime tomorrow?"

With my head still throbbing, I said, "Oh my God, yes, Jeff . . . I'm not well." He laughed so loud I had to move the phone away from my ear. And then I slept for over fifteen hours, before waking up on Tuesday morning feeling stoked.

Questus was headquartered in Tiburon, California, an affluent small town incorporated in Marin County, nestled on Tiburon Peninsula and surrounded on three sides by the San Francisco Bay. An earthen finger pointing accusatorily at shrubby Angel Island opposite the idyllic bayside tourist haven of Sausalito. Questus also ran a tiny satellite office in New York City, which just sounded cool. I imagined telling people I had "to fly out to our New York office for a huge presentation" like Lee Clow or Hal Riney. The agency was housed in a complex of one-story, light-blue buildings wrapped with white decking and nested in an ancient grove of eucalyptus trees. I distinguished the correct suite, breezed into the lobby, and announced my arrival.

His enormous ears detecting my voice, Jeff charged down the hall from his office and enveloped me in a tooth-paste-tube hug. Out of the corner of my eye, I detected a conservatively attired, handsome man approaching with an awkward smile. Once I got my feet back on the ground, I pivoted, reached out, grasped and shook emphatically the man's outstretched hand. "Nice to meet you, Jordan," I told him. "I'm Joey."

"Yeah, dude. I know," he said, his facial expression and posture slipping, voice tapering. "I was with you all weekend in Vegas."

In seven well-dressed words that had showed up at the wrong party, my employment prospects went from promising to dead on arrival. Jeff hemmed with laughter like Jordan had stepped on a rake. Lucky for me, Jordan's sense of humor was stronger than my addled memory.

Jeff (Rosie if you're a friend) served as the agency's research director, while Jordan was the creative director. They led a team of five talented professionals. Rosie was a pioneer in the business applications of online usability research, a field of study that cut across the curriculum from statistics to sociology to cognitive science and used fancy technology to isolate, gather, harvest, sort, group, count, measure, and store every bit and byte related to the media consumer's interactive experience. Every number meant something. Browsing clicks, confirming and purchasing double clicks, microseconds parked in each metered space, walk-ons, walk-outs, comebacks, gross revenue. The Disney Corporation was a Questus client, retaining Rosie to conduct usability studies of its magic mountain of media traffic data. I was immediately sold on Jeff. I can sell smart. I learned a lot about Jordan. In addition to earning his bachelor of arts degree in history from the University of Vermont, he had studied art at the Academy of Art in San Francisco. Jordan had the unique ability to calibrate the shapes, concepts, and colors of his artistry to the objectives of corporate clients, which kept the sudden wannabe graphic designers from pulling on the white coat of Dr. Frankenstein to cobble together some disassembled version of life with graveyard parts. Jordan's biggest client was Suzuki Motorcycles of America; the relationship had been consummated a few months earlier. Motorcycles! Fucking motorcycles. I could sell this dude, too.

As I listened to and observed both men, a rare opportunity revealed itself, like finding money on the street or hitting a straight flush on the flop. These guys were good. Talented. Big brains. Survived an industrial recession. Fortune 400 clients. Questus was an undervalued company, good for an annual triple-decimal pop in increased revenue and profit percentages, with the potential to increase tenfold the company's revenue in half the time elapsed since it was founded. Making the partners rich in the process. I felt transported to Steve Wozniak's garage in the seventies, like I was listening to some bespectacled guy in a black turtleneck predict the orbit of the recently discovered planet Apple. I decided to go all in. But only as an owner. I bragged about millions of dollars of revenue increases during my tenure at BI, an agency similar to Questus in size and services. I embellished in legitimate detail my experience breeding relationships with corporate whales in the financial industry. I closed by explaining that if I was going to turn down job offers with stock options and big salaries, I wanted the opportunity to share in the rewards. I wanted equity. I left exhausted, but optimistic. Didn't sleep well that night.

After a slow-drip twenty-four-hour period, I answered my phone on the first ring and heard Jeff offer me an equity partnership at the same salary they paid themselves with any additional income to be calculated by meeting performance objectives of a built-in compensation structure, priming the pump for huge Joey bonuses. Jeff reminded me, "We eat what we kill around here, Joey, so if you don't kill, you don't eat," adding, "You'll never outsell me." Such a dude thing to say. Game on, Rosie! I accepted immediately and ended the call quickly, shuddering as morphine heat ran up the back of my legs to flood my brain and chest cavity. The capitalist orgasm. A hit I had craved for months. Almost as good as the sex I was about to have. The salary would more than meet my needs while the bonus structure generated compounding income unallocated to any overhead expenses and therefore available for investment and strong returns. Once my bonuses were factored into my salary, my hourly rate effectively rose 400 percent per hour. As if there were now four cloned employed Joeys. I liked the sound of Joey—how can you take yourself seriously when your name is Joey.

It was also at this moment, where I decided to go by the name Joey instead of Joseph. How can you take yourself seriously you're your name is Joey. Something beyond survival. Life engorged.

I was a new partner at Questus. Good for me. My meteoric rise to the company's executive ranks was announced at the next morning's staff meeting. The five facial expressions—angry, disappointed, indifferent, perplexed, and disgusted—implied that a few perceived me as undeserving. I wondered whether my fly was open. Jen, the head of client services, had attended the University of Vermont with Jeff and Jordan and since 1999 managed all of the company's creative projects, timelines, and visual design meetings. She was intelligent, soft-spoken, good at her job, and sourpuss unimpressed with the new management. Laura, educated at Baylor University and blessed with high levels of emotional and social intelligence, had worked on Jeff's team as a researcher since 2002 and appeared equally disappointed. Glen was Jeff's other research associate. He had graduated from Boston College and still presented identical to his freshman ID photo: white Polo shirt, college cap, khaki pants, flip-flops, cloth belt with birds on it. Glen appeared not to dislike me. Twenty-two years old and a recent graduate from Lehigh University, Kerry handled project management, and was the only person in the office unable to reconcile her nerves with the bass thunder of Jeff's voice and physical presence. She smiled a lot. Linda served as part-time controller working two days a week. Linda fired off a clip of prosecutorial questions regarding my book of client contacts, number of executed six-figure contracts, annual revenue stats, and curve trajectories.

Rosie wanted me to sell both advertising and market research services. I had some professional league experience in the former, but found myself embarrassingly unqualified to pitch the latter, manning the mound like some floppy-armed, half-inflated flexible tube man. Market research is an organized set of rules and practices applied to gather information about target markets, to master narratives of buyer biographies and purchasing demographics, incorporating all of the language and concepts formally taught in the STEAM classes I either failed or failed to take: science, technology, engineering, arts, and mathematics. Rosie left bundles of market research reports on my desk, texts tightly woven with specialized discourse, anthill numbers, conceptual models and diagrams, probability and statistics, sociology, psychology, logic, cognitive science, biology, and anthropology. "Let me know if you have any questions, Joey." Sure thing, Jeff. What's *regression analysis*? How does *falsifiability null* a *hypothesis*? Do *top box numbers* refer to box tops? Can you use *semiotics* in a sentence? Why is *hermeneutics* spelled with five vowels?

Out of fear and loathing, I began to read market research in all of its forms. As if being chased. But after a few weeks of oppressive study, all I could think about was the revenue I was not raising. So I decided to wing it. I called Brett, the MTV executive from Scotty's bachelor party with whom I had bonded again at the wedding in St. John, and asked for some face time with a few of his research teams who worked behind the scenes at MTV, VH1, and Nickelodeon. Brett landed us meetings within the next two weeks. A half dozen research professionals based out of the East Coast clicked yes on our calendar invite and sacrificed a small block of their valuable workday to meet with Jeff Edison and Joey Tesla. All of us would receive increasingly frequent periodic reminder windows on our monitors of the big day. You could feel the excitement.

Thirteen days later, Rosie and I flew to New York City and checked into a tiny litter box of a hotel room on the lower West Side the night before our presentations, trading additional preparation time for a pre-victory celebration of our initiative and intellectual prowess with Jeff's old fraternity buddy, Billy Beer. Great dude. The mind of Manhattan flexes on stimulated energy, stays awake for days, tosses and turns all night, and has the power to short out any sense of reality in its own private dance. For the next six hours we were Jake and Elwood on a mission from God, starring in musical numbers with attractive performers just out of reach of pursuing consequences.

As we approached the lobby of our hotel six hours prior to our first meeting at MTV, I saw a small bodega from which I wanted something to counter our chances of alcohol poisoning. I told Rosie to wait for me. While cradling two swaddled three-pound burritos and a huge smile, I jogged back to our hotel and saw Rosie leaning on a couch in the lobby. Raising the twins above my shoulders so Rosie could appreciate my binge-ending stroke of late-night genius, I accelerated up the walkway until the pristine, thick tempered glass panel of the lobby door flattened me like a cartoon character. My face struck the door first, the impact hammering the shrapnel of my designer frames into my left eyebrow. Then the rest of me. Vertical then horizontal. Laughing on my back with a wailing burrito in each hand. An elongating bloodworm crawled down the left side of my drunken head. Rosie laughed so hard his knees gave out. Hotel security was more subdued—and less impressed: "Go sleep it off, sir." Rosie obtained from the doorman some first aid supplies and back at the room may have attempted to sew up the gash on my eyebrow. We don't remember. The dynamic duo awoke four hours later experiencing competing currents of exhilaration and nausea. Drank lots of water and took long therapy showers. Changed the dressing on my still throbbing wound. Large tip for the horrified housekeeper.

We had two meetings booked with Viacom executives, one with MTV at 10 a.m. and one with VH1 at 2 p.m. I assured Rosie I had memorized every slide, each word of copy, even my crack-filling commentary and humorous improvisations. We arrived with time to spare at skyscraping 1515 Broadway, where the Viacom offices were housed, smack dab in the heart of Times Square, the city's hazy, techno-thumping, steel-and-concrete plaza. We took the elevator to the MTV offices on the thirty-sixth floor and were escorted to a media-savvy conference room with walls and ceilings affixed with Voice of God speakers, projector-screen-sized digital displays covering three walls, and high-backed padded leather executive chairs. Like a megachurch or man cave. Or a Buffalo Wild Wings.

Three professionally attired and groomed women were encamped at the conference room table. As we hooked up our laptops, we tooted small talk: "So do you guys live in Manhattan? Bet you never get tired of the view." "Does MTV stand for something?" "Do any of you know Martha Quinn?" The woman sitting between the other two, obviously the leader, who by virtue of her lean height, prominent nose, and Oreo eyes possessed an avian quality, looked up from her computer and chirped, "I have a hard stop at 11 a.m.," which in business parlance translates to "Shut the fuck up and get on with it already!" I stepped up and delivered my portion of our presentation, getting through about half of my slides and copy—even my best jokes—without any major breaks and falls. But about the time I was going to hand the baton to Rosie, Ms. Hard Stop at 11 a.m. dropped and raised her head. "How does your regression analysis measure the independent variables you showed in your last case study?" Ouch. It was only one second of vacuum silence, but I must have looked like a rat caught in a spotlight because she promptly turned to focus expectantly on Rosie.

The quality of his reply raised the temperature of their expectations, and the room seemed to warm up a bit. I felt like an unclaimed bag at the airport. When I froze again after her next question about small sample populations, overreaching extrapolations, and failures to account for standard deviations, she reverted to mockery: "So your job is basically done here, huh, Joey?" Which translates to "You idiot poseur. I hate you.

And you're named after a baby kangaroo." Someone must have taught her that an insult inflicted more damage when you toe-tagged the target's name. Well played, madam. Rosie adeptly answered her questions, but it no longer mattered. *Excuse me. One of my testicles is caught in your talons. Yup. That's it. Thank you. We'll be on our way.* They had no interest in another Beavis and Butthead. On the elevator, I told Rosie I wasn't going to present at the next meeting. He understood completely. Probably relieved.

At our 2 p.m. meeting with VH1, the scene repeated itself, but with one fewer actor lying in wait in an empty conference room hiding behind propped screens like a sniper. Two heads briefly popped up in greeting, instructing us to set up. Rosie tossed off a crippled quip about market research being easier than connecting cables from our computers to the access ports. Clicking keyboard crickets. A long minute later, Jeff introduced us and asked the panel to tell us a little bit about their roles and duties at VH1. "My name is Maura," announced the alpha, "and I lead the quantitative research group here. This is my colleague, Jody."

Rosie leaped into his presentation, "Well, Laura, at Questus we believe research is the . . ."

Maura stopped him immediately with a hand and interrupted, "Excuse me," before annunciating very slowly, "My name is Maura." As in *moron*. Or *muff*.

"God, with ears this big, you'd think I'd be able to hear you the first time!" Rosie exclaimed. Or at least avoid tripping over them. I made the moment even more unsatisfying by chortling my support, loudly and unaccompanied,

tapping the impromptu humiliation of being caught performing an off-key *a cappella* solo of a favorite song in a crowded
vehicle during a momentary lapse of the radio signal. Our faces felt scorched. Then it got worse. Balls dropped and kicked.
We got cancelled. Afterward, I looked at Jeff and lamented,
"Dude, we could have told Maura she was adopted and had a
better day. That's it for me, man."

Chapter 21

## Joey Questus
### (2003-2006)

I immediately disregarded the high-volume shotgun sales strategy that built Questus. Although casting wide nets to capture schools of prey worked for king crab fisherman, too much of my irreplaceable contact time got lost in the logistics of individual meetings, throat-drying door-to-door canned sales presentations, redundant process communications, asscovering documentation, and the limits of a twelve-hour workday. To me, it made more sense to hunt whales, Moby Dick or otherwise. My target companies had familiar brand names, obese media service budgets, and a genuine desire to explore the financial frontiers of virtual space. The executive decision-makers of the mid-2000s, educated by the 2001 crash, were industry savvy and technically adept, and demanded the highest level of expertise, service, and exponential returns for their investment dollar. My job was to get Questus into each corporate whale's bidding pool, the finite group of potential brands invited by that corporation to solicit their products and services through a formal written instrument. The term for these solicitations is a *request for proposal* (RFP).

The response to an RFP is not a glossy pamphlet riddled with marketing bullets or a facile, seizure-inducing PowerPoint presentation. You don't knock it out the night before like some grade school book report. No obvious embellishments, half disclosures, or abstract generalizations. No cheap sales talk. Instead, this carefully crafted, logically presented, word-processed sales instrument reads like a socioeconomic industrial ethnography, with expert biographies and verifiable sources and successes, framed by the agency's vision and capacity to meet the client's business objectives. Sounds impressive, huh? Hundreds of hours can go into what resembles an audition on paper, a chaptered story that educates, inspires, analyzes, predicts, qualifies, quantifies, and argues that your agency is the best fit for the requesting company. Through our proposal, we disclosed every relevant fact regarding our corporate information and history, including such granular detail as how many military hires we had (or would hire) and the specific education and experience held by each team member, proving our financial strength to alleviate any liquidity or bankruptcy concerns, articulate our technical capabilities and limits, and provide specific product information and legitimate customer references. This all made for hours of required reading.

If the RFP leads to the formation and execution of a contract between the companies, a new set of processes begins as the brand interacts with the agency. Throughout the research and development phase, the agency shares perspectives related to meter-running process, communication, and creative development and design sessions, with different actors allocated to specialized tasks: making rounds of revisions, allocating resources, and controlling and balancing budgets. Project people would monitor the system for balance and productivity, and compliance with creative objectives and financial controls. The account leads oversaw all external client management, as well as the internal communication and oversight within the agency. I acted as concierge and cruise director to an array of conflicting stakeholders, critics, and egos in a network in which each contact impacted the output of the entire system. Butterfly effects and chaos theory kind of stuff.

I had hoped to start my Questus career with some early wins to cheer my legitimacy. Instead, we placed runner-up on a Reuters World News RFP because of our perceived incapacity to handle such a massive project. Had we won either of the next two RFPs I convinced my partners to submit, the resulting work and income would have justified my salary, my equity interest, and the substantial resources we invested in reaching out to these iconic companies. Let's get back to the booth.

*Well, Bob . . . The first quarter is in the books, and Questus looks as flat and uninspiring as any professional league team I've covered in my career. Late in the period,*

*their new franchise player, Joey Disappointment, went 0-3 on*
*some very makeable baskets. I heard booing at the buzzer.*

Bricking my first trio of costly and laborious RFPs in
the first six months left me predictably shaken and discour-
aged, a potentially job-ending performance problem if Jeff
and Jordan decided to pull me. Jen continued to argue to Jeff
and Jordan for my expulsion while twice a week I would feel
Linda's little word fists punching me in the face: "I thought
you sold millions at your last agency. All I see is expenses!"
No snappy comeback for that. Something was missing. I convinced my partners we needed the expertise of a full-time
account director. Fortunately, the woman I had in mind for the
job was available. Questus hired Esther away from her agency
(the technical term is "poached") a few weeks later to serve as
our newest account director. Esther's first task was to manage
the plesiosaur RFP I had dragged in with my big mouth. Nip-
pon Telegraph and Telephone (NT&T), Japan's largest
telecommunications conglomerate, had recently purchased a
company in the United States for billions of dollars and intended to invest more than a million dollars to completely
redesign its online advertising platforms. With Esther leading
from the front, we won the deal, and NT&T became our first
seven-figure client. The first of many, it turned out. Jeff and
Jordan were ecstatic. No parades, but I felt vindicated.

More companies hired us. We broke the multimillion-
dollar annual revenue milestone. Linda stopped poking pins in
her Joey Voodoo doll. But there was no time for anyone to
celebrate, no Corona lime vacations, no visit to Cannes just
yet, as each lucrative contract carried a trailer load of sharp

and weighty legal performance obligations, requiring a larger roster of hungry artists, technologists, and business experts to handle all of the labor. Overhead costs split like stock. Our success attracted to our team a supremely talented artist and reincarnation of Pericles we called JW, with whom Esther had worked on the Apple account at her former agency. By the end of 2004, we had grossed our highest revenue figures in the company's history. But we had ten on the team now, and when the costs of the new hires and failed proposals were factored in, our total expenses exceeded net revenue.

Outgrowing our office suite and too big to fail, Questus relocated its headquarters to a four-square-block neighborhood in San Francisco referred to in the industry as the Agency Gulch, requiring a new lease, a security deposit, first month's rent, insurance, moving costs, service activation, furniture and hardware expenses, and countless other overhead-raising annoyances. Jeff and Jordan seemed excited about our growth, but it must have appeared to the rest of the team like we had taken a step too far. We suffered the tension between caution—the better-looking sister of fear, which can result in stagnation—and ambition, which tends to overreach and can lead to extinction. But it may be through these competing forces between opposite poles that growth emerges.

After a few weeks of bone-softening anxiety, I received a call from one of our clients reporting that Verizon was about to invite RFPs to redesign the company's web presence, and that out of respect for the quality of our work he had referred our agency to the multibillion-dollar corporation for the twelfth and final spot on its RFP roster. The news was so good I thought he was sticking it to me. I kept the expectation to myself, not wanting to play some sick joke mocking the talent and hopes of the team. Verizon's RFP arrived a few days later. Still skeptical, I reviewed it carefully. It was real. Holy shit! Now we had to get to work! Verizon had committed to transmogrifying its image from a stodgy old telecommunications corporation to a hipper, younger brand capable of appealing to a new digital audience. Questus was the last company in the door, forced to sit at the far end of the table in accommodating mismatched chairs, but we made it into the room. We made the playoffs.

We launched into campaign mode, our seasoned squad executing the same drills and plays that had gotten us to this point, putting in fourteen-hour days for the next three weeks developing a strategy and creative treatment for Verizon. Like in the NCAA Basketball Tournament, your initial goal in the RFP process is to make the final four agencies for consideration. In this case, each of those four would receive a personal day-long first date with Verizon's chemistry-check team before the ideal mate would be selected. Questus made the cut.

The timing was perfect. The physical space occupied by Questus modeled the same sets crafted by our industry to digitally depict the awesomeness of what we did: twenty-foot ceilings, majestic windows, romantic exposed-brick walls, a glass-walled incubator conference room and executive offices, all situated around a small soccer field of tactically shifting creative and research team pods known as "the floor," the same term used in stock trading, phone sales, car dealerships, and sporting events. Where only the talent was allowed. The administrators were appropriately relegated to the periphery. Jordan had the corner office, Linda had the middle, and I was on the end (Rosie was now in our New York office). The company appeared larger and more formidable than it was.

Jordan and JW were the starting pitchers, with thirteen spectators crammed into our dugout conference room. Both started strong, and neither gave up any hits. The Verizon audience appeared riveted to the sensory-ripe language and images, the integrated overlays of music and narration. They turned off their cell phones. A week later, I received a call from Kyme, one of the Verizon executives with whom I had worked closely over the past month. "We're awarding the deal to Questus," she stated, "but if you have a daughter one day, you have to name her after me." "Done and done!" I said. Kyme was a cool name. And if it got me the account, so was Gertrude. Kyme and I are still friends to this day.

Questus executed a master service agreement (MSA) with Verizon that broke down to the micron our tangible legal obligations attached to every gold brick of Verizon's service fees, such as how many teammates would work on each segment of each phase of the master project; the hourly billing rate of each expert; the integrated hourly rate for work completed by teams formed for specific tasks; language attempting to quantify quality and satisfaction; extraneous and miscellaneous expenses; and legal, accounting, and administrative service fees. Calibrated each day. Compounded every hour. We were partnered with Verizon's Broadband division, which streamed exclusive content through a proprietary fiberoptic network that included joint ventures with musical artists such as Gwen Stefani, Akon, Jill Scott, and Justin Timberlake, to name a few. Questus was soon billing Verizon millions of dollars. Our teams were now on planes weekly, flying to client meetings all over New York City and Basking Ridge, New Jersey, the headquarters of Verizon. We continued poaching brilliant creative, research, and client services talent from competing agencies, growing to over forty-three employees in eighteen months.

I became a regular on the advertising circuit. Attended quarterly pleasure-packed iMedia Summit weekends where every Who from Whoville gathered for well-compensated, invitation-only networking events, keynotes, creative presentations, technical tutorials, and celebrations of cool campaigns. My individual purpose, however, was to broadcast my own personal brand to industry friends, and to be seen, heard, overheard, recognized, touched, and hugged—to become the implied discussion or the direct object of everyone else's sentences. Attract and hold on to attention. Become massive. Be Joey Huge.

The February 2006 iMedia Summit was hosted at the Camelback Resort in raisin bran Scottsdale, Arizona. "Checking in? Yes, Joey Verizon! Welcome! Yes, sir, your manicure appointment is set for 4:30. Great weather you're having. Have you been working out? May I fluff your pillows?" We pretend to star in our own commercials, shop excitedly, dress for dinner, rotate jewelry, schedule massages, sit patiently for haircuts and pampering nail services, dab on pheromone colognes and perfumes, pose poolside, in restaurants, on golf courses, in conference rooms and ballrooms, and smile in front of mirrors with people who look as good as we do.

As I reclined in the resort's effeminate lumbar-supporting spa chair pondering my next publicity stunt, my right hand the center of attention, the manicurist asked whether the thirty-eight-year-old man preferred a buff or a coating. "Black nail polish, please." Like Johnny Depp. Dave Navarro. Or Herman Munster. My industry deserved credit for promoting the silly science of infinite subtractive shades of black and white pitched by cosmetics and paint manufacturers. Jet. Obsidian. Onyx. Vanta. Ghost. Smoke. Navajo. Snow. Each sold separately. Collect them all. *I'll take Jet, please.*

I decided I would never again wear anyone's employment uniform, whether it was cheap screen-printed pizza parlor T-shirts, gazpacho-stained tuxedos, or hand-stitched cashmere Italian suits. I wanted my clothing and accessories to shout exactly who I was. A rocker who can't play an instrument. Vampire executive. Aging motorcycle pirate. That evening's costume consisted of a pair of perfectly distressed jeans, four mutant power rings, a secret agent watch, and my latest douche couture: a replica of a jacket worn by Shane MacGowan, lead singer of the '80s Irish punk band The Pogues, hand-stitched and adorned with a black button lattice common on band uniforms, a style traceable to the Middle Ages when military bands marched with infantries to provide guidance and inspiration on the battlefield. The jacket brought together my grease-black nails and eyeliner, a Welterweight white belt, and stiff, heightening jack boots. Flamboyant as a Molotov cocktail. Subtle as a car bomb. Some talented former girlfriend could have written a hit song about me as I high-stepped into the opening cocktail party twirling my baton to an adoring mirror. Joey Reflection.

Side effects of regular Summit attendance include liver damage, hangovers, large credit card bills, and enhanced Frequent Flyer status. These realities are bolstered by the promises of new business leads and tons of scheduled entertainment. That's where Joey Swizzle Stick came in. Time to crack some ice and tell some jokes—all part of the show. Unlike any actual work, however, my first order of duty was the Sunday-night cocktail party that always started at 6 p.m. On the dot.

## Chapter 22

## Debbie Dumont
(2006-2010)

By 2006, our team had grown to over fifty people, requiring key hires in our client services department to manage the ever-growing flow of communications between creative teams, strategists, social media technologists, and antsy business executives. It was during this period that Rebecca (our new account director on the Verizon business) hired twenty-seven-year-old Debbie Tung as one of our account team members. Debbie and I would marry four years later, but not until I spent the first two years cultivating her disappointment and perfectly framed ridicule. Her dislike of my persona was irresistible.

Debbie was of Chinese ethnicity and raised in a happy and intact patriarchal family. Thirteen years younger. Bicultural. Multilingual. Taller. More beautiful. Honorable. Respected. Cared about *other* people. Hated tattoos. Business marketing degree from the University of Texas. Traveled the world. Unburdened with baggage. Few previous romances. No embarrassing alcohol or drug exploits. Or burned bridges. Never fired. Honorable and trustworthy. Respected and admired. Close to a family who may dislike me based on all of the above.

I was everything Debbie was not and did not want. Radiohead's "Creep." Moreover, Debbie was in a relationship and technically my employee, producing a slew of cultural and legal taboos. For nearly the first two years of our work life together, my ego attempted to repress every thought of an impossible future, and if possible, sabotage any prospect of a future together. While most men make every effort to apply layers of their best behavior early on in the relationship, I showed Debbie repeated live recordings of my least attractive seasons and security camera footage of how I act when I believe nobody is looking.

I introduced myself to Debbie at a meeting with Verizon, thinking she was an employee of the telco company. And she immediately corrected me with a smile: "I am on your team, Joey. Today is my first day." I was so preoccupied with all things Joey that I was inexcusably unaware of the many new hires. And over the next two years, I displayed a Rocky Horror Picture Show-level performance that included superficial speed dating with too many women in multiple cities, fraternal buffoonery, squads of vices, scads of insecurities, and motorcycle wheelies down North Point Street in front of our ad agency (which got me arrested once). I showed her exactly who I was. Or who I thought I was, anyway.

Verizon invited Questus to construct a technology-based virtual experience for the after-hours parties at the upcoming forty-ninth Annual Grammy Awards in Los Angeles that included a digital red carpet and social media conversations broadcasted in real time. Questus worked behind the scenes, devoting months to planning and schematics, weeks to constructing and honing systems, days to logistics and double-checks, and hours to readiness, all leading to the firing of the starter pistol the second the awards show ended. The day before the event, I rode to the airport with Debbie in our expensed town car, delaying our arrival after stops at Gucci to pick up my suit and Ted Baker to pick up my shoes. My personal shopping steward, Sebastian from the Fifth Avenue store in New York, assisted me in selecting an ivory jacket complemented by coal-black slacks, each with contrasting pinstripes, an opal shirt, a corn silk ascot, and shadow nails and eyeliner. Loud. Even for the Grammys. Hoped to get confused for a nominee (one can always hope). Debbie was speechless. Obviously more amused than impressed, she just laughed. We arrived at the Roosevelt Hotel on Hollywood Boulevard twenty-four hours before our limousine was scheduled to take our party of fifteen to the Grammys. The women and I had salon appointments the next morning. The Grammys began at 7 p.m.

Our elongated, trashy white Hummer limousine arrived wedding dress pregnant and ashamed, each broadside bunted with a ten-digit phone number advertising hard ride rental access. Hardly the upscale luxury vehicle I was promised. I consoled my ego by anticipating the fantasy moment of our arrival, sliding feet first out the opened door, the brief crouch, slow extension to my full, stiff height while buttoning my stylish jacket, capped by calmly gazing at my surroundings through crazy-straw sunglasses with a condescending smile.

In reality, event security would not allow our albino Death Star within a half mile of the venue. We could have unloaded closer driving a ticking U-Haul full of fertilizer. We walked the final leg in the afternoon heat and arrived through monitored side service entrances before being steered into the dusty maze-ways that allowed for movement of personnel and equipment while preventing access to the showered and primped VIP sections.

We were not even to be included among the many millions of viewers, as no televisions were installed in the highly secure reception zone where our after-hours booth and swag were staged. We heard laughter and applause for hours. Sat at a card table and talked about our day. Shared compliments about my suit. We ate some snacks from a vending machine. When the show ended, we cleaned up our candy wrappers and Styrofoam cups and leaped into action. Verizon's digital red carpet was a big hit. We spent hours taking pictures in front of a green screen, sent out social media posts, and socialized with hundreds of our newest friends. After midnight, our limo wedged itself into a Carl's Jr. drive-through so I could buy a dozen Western Bacon Cheeseburgers. Back at the Roosevelt Hotel, we managed to smile our way into a tub-thumping, celebrity-populated party a few doors down from our collective suites. Within ten minutes, a

puffy, drippy P. Diddy approached and told Debbie to meet
him at his room at 2 a.m. He's still waiting. Apparently, cen-
timillionaires need regular reminders of the things they will
never be able to afford. Every time I returned home from the
streets of Hollywood, I took an extra shower.

***

Dad's health problems seeped into my life once again. While
in Marina Del Rey, Dad's sugar habit had begun demanding
blood payments in the form of Type 2 diabetes. He ignored
his diagnosed low insulin levels, allowed the disease to erode
his internal systems and organs, and accelerated the process
by downing horse droppings of apple fritters and spunky
frosted long johns, gallon jugs of fruit syrup mixed with water, candy bar stents, gut bombs of fatty, high-sodium
processed foods, buttered coffee, and as much wine as anyone
would buy him. By the time Dad moved back to Sonoma
County in 2000, his endocrine system had dishonorably dis-
charged thirty pounds of ballasting fat, muscle, and bone
density and lopped twenty years off his lifespan. Over the
next six years, his escalating neuropathy erased all vision in
his left eye and dimmed the right. He acquired a limp. Suffered drenching flop sweats, congestive heart failure, and
kidney damage. By the time he began injecting insulin, the
disease had already played itself out. Dad continued to work
and devoted his free time to racing around Sonoma County in
a heavily leveraged red convertible Mazda Miata, wearing a
floppy sun hat like Meryl Streep.

In the late summer of 2006, Paul and I received a call from Sutter Hospital that Dad had fallen in his Santa Rosa apartment, suffering a number of significant injuries, some predictable, others more difficult to explain. Dad broke his left shoulder and a few ribs. Blackened the left side of his face. Bruises and minor sprains. He also suffered a gaping wound encompassing the larger toes of his left foot that exposed the inner fascia, ligaments, and bones as if some maniac had gouged it with a claw hammer. A month later, the doctors performed a partial amputation, resulting in a smooth, stumpy half foot and shortened pink leg that over time bent back full flamingo. Dad qualified for permanent disability. He would never work again. The Miata was sold. Sugar has cost more American lives and treasure than tobacco.

On a more positive note, Stevie called and told me he was coming out for a week's visit in February of 2007. Paul and I were thrilled to spend time with him. We watched sports. Ate his favorite foods. He especially enjoyed the Cliff House. We shopped and played video games. Purchased gallons of coffee-based products. Stevie sat grinning through one of Paul's legal writing class lectures at Golden Gate University. We were sad to watch him pass through security at the airport when he flew back to Minnesota. A few weeks later, Stevie called me again, excitedly informing me that he was *moving out* to San Francisco, provided he could bunk with me until he was able to establish employment and housing. I was surprised but happy to oblige. After nearly twenty years of involuntary distance, we all had time and space to be together, and I could afford to support him as long as he needed the help. On April 1, 2007, Stevie stuffed his bags into a blue shuttle van outside a dingy hotel off Highway 52, kissed Mom goodbye, and flew out again to San Francisco. On the way home from the airport, we celebrated at a roach coach. Picked up some speakers at the Apple store in Burlingame. Smoked a bunch of weed and watched a lot of Seinfeld. We had a blast. I always treated my time with Stevie like it was circumscribed. I knew he wouldn't make it to old age. His liver alone would take him out.

On April 10, 2007, Stevie visited Questus and went out to lunch with the team at the Hard Rock Cafe at Pier 39. Sometime after 2 p.m., he headed back to my Franklin Street apartment to relax. I told him we would order some pizza and hang out all night after I returned from a motorcycle ride up the coast. We hugged it out. Told each other we loved one another. Arriving home a few hours later, I expected to see Stevie on my couch watching TV. Instead, the apartment was silent. I shouted his name. Silence.

The bathroom door was closed. I knocked. Silence. I kicked open the door with my boot to discover Stevie's motionless body floating face down in the bathtub, bloated purple and blue like a giant berry. An aerosol can was perched on the salmon-colored sink. I screamed as loud as I ever have as my arms pierced the narrow canals around his buoyant body. I somehow managed to haul his two-hundred-pound mass over the edge of the tub, the skin of his lifeless feet slapping the porcelain floor, my T-shirt quickly saturated by the squeeze of tepid bath water released from his curly dark hair against my chest. I dragged his dead weight into the hardwood hallway, where I sat him down between my legs and roared again like a wounded animal. Hands shaking, I fumbled for the cell phone enveloped within my riding jacket and dialed 9-1-1. I don't remember a single word of the call. I laid him on his back and began pumping his heart, hand over hand with locked elbows, then pinched his nose and placed my mouth over his, tasting Tums and wine as I attempted to blow life back into his flooded lungs, his chest expanding and contracting like a blowfish. He was as cold as baloney.

My front door was thrown open by paramedics, three deep, reaching for their gear while ordering me away from the beached body before they heaved it from the hallway to the bedroom where they began to triage. Chest pads with kite-tail wires, cylinder-shaped pumps, an oversized plastic mouthpiece, mechanized hisses and beeps, and the crinkle of opening wrappers became the only sounds in the room. As if on cue, two police officers, a male and a female, walked calmly through the open door into my home and immediately commenced their by-the-book investigation by questioning the most proximate eyewitness. They employed the tired good cop / bad cop routine.

One of them asked, "Why is this man naked?"

I answered, "Do you bathe in your clothes, asshole?"

I disengaged and began moving toward the hectic bedroom, prompting the male officer to place his open hand on my chest. It felt like a starfish.

"You are not allowed in there, sir. This is a crime scene."

"Are you fucking kidding me?"

"Sir, do not make this any more difficult for yourself. You need to sit and talk with us."

It was not until I descended to my couch that I remembered that my full riding leathers and high-buckled racing boots made me look like one of the Village People, my mind only now entertaining the range of inferences elicited by the facts thus far observable to San Francisco law enforcement. Good Cop asked me what had happened.

I took a deep breath and slowly released it, pausing before taking the next, constructing in my head a sentence capable of summarizing the plot and essential actors for a skeptical audience. Just the Facts Joey.

"I returned to my home from a motorcycle ride and found my little brother dead in the bathtub."

The officers appeared to shrink, almost relax, before apologizing.

"Oh, we are sorry, sir. We were investigating a possible murder scene. You are free to go see your brother."

As I entered the bedroom, the actions of the paramedics had lost their prior efficient urgency. The body was still. Ignoring us. The leader, half my age, turned to me with a resigned facial expression, his brow sweaty.

"Sir, why did you say he was gone when we got here?"

"Because I could no longer feel him."

"Say your last goodbyes please."

I knelt over his cold, damp discarded vessel and talked to it like a speaker phone. "I love you so much, little buddy. I'm sorry the world was so hard for you." I ran out of words. Collapsing, I sobbed over a body that resembled less with each viewing my brother. I left the bedroom and called Paul in Hawaii, where he was coaching a gymnastics meet. He answered right away, interpreted my hysterical sentences and peppered me with factual questions. Eventually I said, "You gotta call Mom, dude . . . I can't hear her wail right now. I just can't do it."

"I got this, Joe. I love you, and this is not your fault. Call Kimmy."

By morning, everyone else in my world would feel some of our family's pain. Fill up my voicemail. A Hard Rock Cafe receipt recovered from his pocket indicated that on the walk home Stevie had gone back to the bar and purchased two glasses of Chardonnay after I left him to go back to work. The bartender was likely the last person to hear him speak. Stevie probably tried to hug him goodbye. I lay in a coma like state on my couch staring at the ceiling. I heard the zipper of the body bag. The coroner presented his business card.

"Call me if you have any questions or concerns with the corpse."

A few days after Stevie's funeral, Paul flew back to California with our two-hundred-twenty-pound puffer fish father, arriving after midnight at the emergency room in Santa Rosa where dutiful medical professionals drained Dad like a used-up waterbed. I flew to Los Angeles to attend the Gwen Stefani friends and family concert with the team. It was comforting to see everyone. I got lots of hugs. But I'll never forget Debbie's personal presence and kindness. Months later, as I was checking out photos from our Verizon music tour with

Rebecca, she pointed to a great photo of me. "Do you notice anything, Joey?"

"I sure do. I got that jacket at John Varvatos . . ."

"Not your clothes, you jackass! The fact that you and Debbie are always sitting next to each other." Rebecca fanned through the pages, pausing periodically to point out images supporting her observation. "When you are done playing around with all your little girlfriends in New York, I think you and Debbie would be a great couple." Debbie and Joey. Joey and Debbie. Debbie Dumont. Mr. and Mrs. Joey Dumont. I couldn't wait to tell Debbie the good news. Just needed to overcome a sky-darkening hail of objections raised by character, cultural conflicts, karma, common sense, better angels, Debbie, her suspicious sisters, her extended family members, her legion of superfriends, her colleagues, her protective, conservative immigrant Chinese parents, and California law. Successful marriages, like all successful personal relationships, require the following load-bearing support structures beyond our primal animal instincts: *love, respect,* and *trust*— in that order, and I lacked all three with Debbie. While love could grow from emotion, trust and respect demanded facts, results, and accountability. Reciprocity. Integrity. Trust and respect kept score on home field jumbotrons. Perhaps if I could show Debbie that she loved me, I could earn back the other two. I had to find out.

A few months later in New York City, our team met at a bar in Korea Town to karaoke our hearts out after another big win. About three o'clock in the morning, drunk and overly confident, I approached a comparatively sober and alert Debbie and announced my courtship campaign and solicitation of her RFP by trivializing what should have been a sparkling memory in her beautiful life.

"So what are we going to do about us?"

Debbie scrunched up her pretty face and said, "What do you mean?"

At this point in every happy-ending rom com, the protagonist reforms a self-immolating comment unheard the first time by the beloved into a similar-sounding, appropriate witty one-liner. *So what are we going to do about breakfast? The shuttle bus? Festivus?* Instead, I threw on some paraphrasing gasoline and flicked my Bic.

"I have feelings for you, and I think you feel the same."

She immediately burst into tears. "You asshole. I take my job seriously, and you're a partner at this agency. I would never date you anyway. You're a pig and sleep with everyone."

Cogent as a slap, her brutally honest and painfully accurate summation made me want her that much more. Good time for an intermission. Locate the blown-off pieces of my face. Regroup. Try again at the hotel.

Later that night, I tripped three more testimonial landmines: "Hey, I'm sorry I made you cry earlier" (an admission of culpability); "I'm not trying to get you into bed" (material misrepresentation); and "We're going to get married and have babies together someday" (lacked foundation, assumed facts not in evidence; plea of insanity).

She said, "Now I just think you're creepy."

But I was correct. I could always tell when a woman liked me based on the quality of the rejection. Apathy could care less. Hate gave a shit. Debbie had a black belt in language arts. Her words mattered. Contained mass, gravitas, and clarity. Could be found in dictionaries and founding documents. Chiseled in stone. Took down and pinned opponents. Debbie didn't lie. She didn't engage in puffery, deflections, gaslighting, shading, slanting, shenanigans, or any other slippery language in the douchebag arsenal, and was therefore resistant to these and all other forms of poisoned or fractured truth. Too honest to cheat or be cheated. Any woman powerful enough to call you out to your face was worth pursuing.

I had some explaining to do. Deprecations. Disclosures. Admissions. Confessions. To earn the most important position in Debbie's life, I told Debbie everything. Honored and adapted to warmer conversational climates: face-to-face discussions, pillow talk, baby talk, family talk, pet names, promises of fidelity, private disclosures, aspirations, hushed signals of evaporating body language. Even the truth. I replaced slick advertisements with PBS documentaries. Mindless chatter with easy listening. Admitted my past, especially the failures. My rank in the pantheon of idiots. The depths of my mine shaft. Somehow, Debbie was able to see me and the man she needed in the same person.

My family was overjoyed with Debbie. The sooner we married the better. My little Mom, after taking an afternoon walk with Debbie through the Fillmore District, got in my face with her pointy little index finger and warned me, "You better be good to her!" My welcome in Austin, Texas, was more tepid. Debbie's wonderfully caring mother cried when she first heard me described over the phone ("Oh, Mei Mei, he is so old!"). Her older sister, an attending pediatric physician at a major hospital, was not impressed with Debbie's Joey Boyfriend action figure, Joey Wrinkles. Her younger sister, also employed in the business of advertising, was equally watchful and protective. The one-year-old niece kept giving me the stink eye (smart little girl). Debbie's enlightened, soft-spoken, genius IBM-engineer father was a perfect gentleman who was as calm as Buddha and welcomed me into his family with a smile and a nod.

Employment law issues had to be addressed. I told Jeff and Jordan I was in love with Debbie. "Debbie?" they asked. "Debbie who? Our Debbie?" I probably deserved that. Jordan immediately called our attorney to report that his imbecilic partner was dating one of our executives. Debbie and I both signed disclosures and waivers enumerated in our anti-sexual-harassment love contract sent over by counsel. I was pumped to have something about our relationship in writing. We married on May 22, 2010, in Mexico in front of a host of loved ones. Best day of my life.

# Chapter 23

---

## Joey Daddy
### (2011-Present)

Kingston Dumont, born in 2011, and Kannon Dumont, born in 2013, are now the center of attention in our slowly expanding life together. Perfect and healthy. Debbie and I catch each other staring at them while they play with their toys. They are tall and thin and strong like Debbie. Powerful. Brilliant. Beautiful. They inherited her compassion and intellect. Communicate in English and Mandarin. They look like both of us. Move like I do. Inherited my attention span. Never stop talking. Fastidious about hair and clothing. They love soccer shoes and looking in the mirror. They jump into our bed too often. Kingston was named after Debbie's hometown in upstate New York, where her memories are as good as she is. Kannon in Buddhism is a bodhisattva, a being prolonging eternal enlightenment to help others in the world. Their middle names honor family. Names we hope to hear for the rest of our lives like favorite songs. Uncle Paul lives down the street. Helps with childcare, baths, and bedtime. Cheers at every event. Spends every holiday with us. The boys used to believe everyone had an Uncle Paul who treated you like the most important person in the world. We are a happy little family.

Our days rise and set with our children. Protecting. Loving. Educating. Kingston and Kannon have attended both private and public Mandarin immersion school since age two, received ongoing professional instruction in humanities, music, visual and language arts, and STEAM education, and participated extensively in organized athletics. They have home access to stacks and shelves of books on any curious subject: *Harry Potter*, *Captain Underpants*, *Diary of a Wimpy Kid*, *Gray's Anatomy*, the *Elements*, classic *Iron Man* and *Avengers* comics, and, with restrictions, the internet. They sing into microphones and strum amplified guitars. Tell jokes. Carry around books in progress. Draw maps. Invent games. Spill paint. Build Legos and paper airplanes. Solve cubes. Watch soccer videos. Ask questions every minute and talk over each other. They have a lot of friends.

A few months before Kingston was born, Dad was informed that his kidneys had shut down. He had two options: hospice or commencement of a three-day-per-week dialysis regimen. Paul bluntly told Dad to forego the oppressive treatment and enjoy his final days. The following day, I sat on the side of his hospital bed and said, "Dad, I would like you to meet my little boy—your grandson."

He said, "Do you really want me to meet him, Joseph?"

"Yeah, dad, I do. I still love you, ya know."

Dad chose to go on dialysis.

On Thanksgiving weekend, Dad got a ride down to San Francisco to visit two-month-old Kingston, who freaked out when we placed him on Grandpa's lap. It was the first time our little boy had ever protested someone else's presence. Smart kid.

Over the holidays, my appendix burst a few hours after I arrived at my childhood home, requiring emergency surgery at one of Rochester's excellent medical centers. The next morning, Paul received a call from the dialysis center that Dad had missed his appointment. Twenty-four hours passed before Paul got Dad on the phone. They agreed to talk the next day. As I recovered from my second surgery, Paul walked into my hospital room after a quiet phone call said, "Dad died last night, Joe."

I don't remember much of what I said, but I do remember saying, "Of course he did . . . We weren't there to take care of him."

Paul just smiled and said, "Are you okay?"

"Yeah. I'll cry later, after I walk out of here. Thanks for taking care of everything, dude. I am obviously not much help." We both laughed. I never cried.

Debbie took the day shifts sitting next to my bed. Paul spent every night shift in the same spot. Nine days later, Paul flew home to arrange for Dad's cremation and deal with his now abandoned apartment and all of his worldly positions. I was able to fly home with Debbie and Kingston the following week. Four months later, the urn containing Dad's ashes were

interned in Mankato, Minnesota, under a tiny stone a few feet
from the graves of his parents. Only immediate family members attended: his twin brother, John, and my Auntie Barbara,
and his sister, Kari, all of whom I love dearly. Dad's small
circle of life. He had no friends. At the short, drizzling cere-
mony, I offered a few positive remarks about my father and
told him I loved him one last time while looking upward. Paul
declined to speak. His way of giving Dad the finger. On the
way to the restaurant, the sun came out, drawing up the rain,
any tears, and most of our memories of my late father.

\*\*\*

While Debbie's personality, upbringing, and accomplishments
primed her for marriage and parenting, Weak Link Joey Cen-
tric required some karmic retooling to cope with the
exponential complexity and great expectations of building a
family. Truant to teacher. Screw-off to coach. Puppet to real
boy. Nothing was simple anymore. Checkers moved to chess.
Astrology graduated to astronomy. Solitaire folded to hold
'em. Long-running family dramas—whether *All in the Family*, *Family Guy*, *Modern Family*, or *Family Feud*—required of
their actors a mastery of space and balance performed in proximity at unimaginable velocities. The challenge of competing
in clusters without colliding. My well-being became condi-
tional. If Debbie and the boys were healthy and happy, so was
I, and conversely, if any one of them was in any type of pain
or distress, I was a mess. My three-generation inner family
circle now included Debbie's parents, sisters, and their fami-

lies residing in Austin, Texas, and my little Mom in Rochester, Minnesota—eighteen people, a stable number until time
reduces our leadership and the next generation swells our
ranks. Enough to fill a lifeboat. Over millions of decisions,
our family evolved into a multistar system. My single-cell
organism somehow evolved into a team of multicellular human beings. Happy to have the help. I've never been so
happy.

When Kingston started preschool in 2014, Debbie and
I took turns with drop-offs and pickups as part of our com-
mutes. I looked forward to these two-minute rides, but I found
the exchanges both sweet and sour. While the thrill of being
reunited each afternoon was intoxicating and joyful, it cut my
heart to wave goodbye to their adorable morning faces as I
drove off to my job. I felt I was going the wrong way. For the
first time in my life, I couldn't have cared less about work. I
was different, or wanted to be. I lost my edge. Puff the Joey
Ego gave way to other joys. I needed some guidance.

***

Nationally recognized for his artistic and ethical contributions
to our industry, John Durham is an adored icon in the world of
advertising and a professor at the University of San Francisco
School of Management. Our first connection at an iMedia
event in 2005 evolved over a decade into friendship. Needing
his advice and a long hug, I invited him to lunch at a little Italian joint he liked near his office. After our beverages arrived,

John looked over at me and spoke softly: "How are you, Joey?"

Rather than volley John's simple informal greeting with a brief positive response such as "Fine, thanks. And you?", I announced to the entire dining room, "I'm getting my ass kicked in the tech space, John—and I fucking hate it! At what point does this kind of failure infect my reputation?"

John took a slow sip from his teacup and smiled. "Well, Joey, nine out of ten start-ups flame out in the first five years, so you have nothing to worry about—yet. In the meantime, the veal parmigiana here is superb." After the server took our orders, John sat back and relaxed his posture, as if he had all the time in the world. "How is Debbie? And how are those beautiful boys of yours?"

I spent most of our remaining time together force-feeding John links of stories about my little boys and their amazing mother as he listened intently. As we wrapped up, John reminded me, "Follow your heart, Joey, just like you did at Questus, and all will be fine." I let him pay for lunch. In hindsight, I believe this discussion with John put me on the path to writing this book.

Fortunately, as my satisfaction in the world of business began to wane, Debbie's corporate success allowed me the time to figure out what I wanted to do with the rest of my life. It now made economic and common sense that Debbie act as the primary wage earner and manage the household, while I would become a stay-at-home dad, handle all pickups and drop-offs at school, assist around the house, be available for doctors' appointments and sick days. I definitely got the better role and the lighter workload. Debbie knew I needed it. She always knew.

At that time, *Curious George* was a major literary figure in our home. Volumes of the beautifully written and illustrated series by H. A. Rey and Margret Rey were among the first books the boys wanted read to them during their squirming toddler days and some of the first books they read on their own. George lived the discovery days of a little boy under the protection of his guardian and primary caregiver, Ted, the man with the yellow hat. Each episode, George's healthy curiosity got him into trouble, requiring the resourceful little monkey to apply newly learned lessons to resolve his challenges relating to a new world.

Like George, my little dudes were instinctively curious, wanting to know about everything they encountered on our short Russian Hill walks. They stopped to smell the colorful flowers bordering the sidewalk, played with ladybugs, beetles, and roly polies, and pointed to shards of glass like they were jewels. They chirped at birds, their tiny, warm fingers skimming every reachable bush, branch, and tree trunk. They waved at cable cars. Moved away from yipping dogs. Never stopped asking questions, demanding that their daddy name the plants and animals and paying for my knowledge with huge smiles and big eyes. They were fascinated by garbage trucks (they thought they were spaceships). Kannon's chubby legs and diaper butt slowed our journeys down comically, requiring an entire half hour for the three of us to small-step the short walk to school. I found myself in no hurry for the first time in years, knowing that this too would pass and wishing that I didn't know that.

# Chapter 24

## Joey Patsy
### (2012-2013)

American douchebags made easy marks. Prancing big-antlered targets. Easily seen coming. It hurts to confess that from 2012 to 2013 I got taken in by not one but two smarmy confidence men whose counterfeit words injured close friends and even my own family. Sucker Joey. Joey the Pinch. Still needing validation from a father figure. The first man attached to me in 2012 and scammed $60,000 in consulting fees from Questus in the months leading up to his arrest and five-year conviction for scamming $21 million from film investors. The other hired me away from Questus to raise talent and funding for a death-spiraling company with a flawed business model that cratered five months later. Both relationships began with promising first dates, moved through grooming and courtship phases, and ended with post-transactional shame and damaging revelations. Our children will require powerful douchebag deflector shields. In case gullibility is genetic.

Daniel Laugher and I met at a media conference at the Mark Hopkins Hotel at the top of Nob Hill on a foggy San Francisco evening. Daniel had enjoyed success as a producer for many hit shows on a major comedy channel. He was in his midsixties, six foot two, and handsome, with a healthy shock of gray hair, a matching goatee, and a Hollywood smile. He dressed, carried himself, and spoke like a successful producer of television shows. Conference goers gathered and sidled up to sit at David's table like we were at the last supper. My elbow jabbed a rack of encroaching ribs. After dinner, blushing, Daniel and I exchanged phone numbers. In parting, he leaned into me, speaking softly: "Joey, I watched your *Naked Brand* documentary and thought it was amazing." I hardly slept that night.

I called David the next day as soon as I walked into my office. He picked up immediately. Like we had never parted. "Joey, I have been thinking about you since I left dinner last night. We are going to do something big here." David dropped A-list names like anvils, informing me of their eagerness to become personally involved in *The Naked Brand* documentary: Jeff Zucker at CNN, Frank Rich, Howard Stern, Bill Maher. He would make some calls. When I picked up Daniel downtown a few weeks later, I received more strokes: "Of course you drive a car like this, Joey. All you ad guys drive cars like this." Ad guy. He called me an Ad Guy. Arriving at the hotel, I handed my key fob and a folded twenty-dollar bill to the valet to park my car within pissing distance.

Over dinner, Daniel told me, "Joey, I only work with people I like; you are hilarious, smart, creative, and really on to something here. I think you and your partners really captured the future of the advertising world with this film." Check, please.

Daniel provided Questus with amazing creative and technical assistance in responding to an important RFP for ASICS. When Daniel stated that we should formalize our relationship, I expected him to propose a figure far beyond our budget range. Instead, he only wanted $20,000 a month and a fair percentage of the spoils on any and all television deals related to *The Naked Brand*. We executed a contract to bring Daniel Laugher on board as a consultant. Set up periodic payments between bank accounts. This was going to be huge!

Over the next few months, in addition to long phone conversations and regular emails, Daniel and I hooked up a few times in LA to sit down with members of his network. He always picked me up from the airport, barely able to field the barrage of speakerphone calls with Hollywood elite related to our project as we sped to some posh cafe or restaurant for me to expense. Many of the face-to-face meetings were arranged at the Beverly Hills Hotel where once I observed Mark Wahlberg sitting in the booth next to us. I heard Dirk Diggler's voice ordering a Spinach salad. Intoxicating. I met a new and different friend of Daniel's each visit, though never the person he had promised. They were all accomplished men and great storytellers with impeccable manners who expressed genuine gratitude for the opportunity to discuss our project over lunch, but it felt like each had been called in at the last minute, and I knew at each hand-grabbing, shoulder-slapping parting I would never hear from any of these people. Joey Who? Never heard of him.

I was relaxing in Hawaii with my family when I answered the phone to hear Daniel's panicky voice explaining he was being investigated by the FBI for his past role as president of Motion Picture Conglomerate, a company that had raised over $20 million to produce five *Pixar*-type productions, including a modern adaptation of *The Wizard of Oz*. But according to the Justice Department, the funds had never reached the intended project. Instead, Daniel and his partner used most of the capital for funding their opulent poseur lifestyles. Daniel confessed his anxiety. Sounded guilty without an admission. He knew my next call would be to Jordan to cut off his consulting fees. He asked for money. It finally dawned on me why Daniel had so much time to hang out with Joey. Everyone else had already given up on him. Cancelled or stood him up on promised meetings scheduled out of embarrassment. Or declined on the spot. Wouldn't return his voicemails. Blocked his emails. Unfriended and blackballed him. The Hollywood Heisman. He was convicted of wire fraud two years later and sentenced to five years in prison.

\*\*\*

I met Tyler Duncan on a first-class flight home from Arizona in June of 2012 that included a few hours on the Sky Harbor tarmac. Tyler projected energy, intelligence, and the confidence of someone who carried inside information. He disclosed his position as CEO of a tech company called Digital Recognition Corporation (DRC), a start-up founded in 2010 powered by cutting-edge proprietary image-recognition software, a concept he came up with during his tenure as chief operating officer for a major singer-songwriter. Tyler explained that the company was originally funded with $24 million raised by a high-profile group of investors, and that the next phase of funding, over $7 million, was forthcoming. The idea was beautiful in its simplicity. DRC found a way to link digital images to products that were sold online. Users clicked, for example, on a celebrity's high-top sneakers to access a tiny pop-up graphic bubble disclosing the designer, manufacturer, price, and distributors. Tyler believed this idea would revolutionize media advertising. His enthusiasm was infectious. We exchanged contact information.

Tyler and I remained in touch over the next year. He visited the agency to present his technology to our executives. He invited Debbie and me to the Critics Choice Awards in Los Angeles, where his image-recognition technology was being featured on the red carpet with selected designers. We hung out with Henry Cavill, the actor who played Superman. Which was super cool. And when Tyler invited us to his son's birthday party in late November 2013, I sensed some sort of proposal was forthcoming. Sure enough, at the party, Tyler asked me to join his executive team as his chief revenue officer (CRO). I was flattered but confused. I could not recall whether I had shared with him that my partners and I were at a crossroads with our agency plan. Events dragged behind the hurtling vehicle of someone else's script.

On further reflection, I was unwilling to face the challenges that had developed at Questus and equally unwilling to investigate DRC and its CEO, and I acted in a fog of willful ignorance and my usual level of arrogance in resigning from the best job I ever had. When I told Tyler I was accepting his offer and looking forward to starting my new position at the beginning of the year, Tyler laughed. "You've never worked at a start-up before, have you? Every day matters, Joey. I need you to start now." I agreed. Apparently losing a month of family time was not a deal-breaker for me.

One of my duties as a CRO was to help DRC design a revenue model that aligned with their technology. Identify customer bases. Price points. Evidence of growth potential and scalability. Publishers like Viacom own online web properties like MTV, VH1, and Nickelodeon. Brands like Nike, Adidas, and McDonald's paid Viacom to advertise through all of their mediums. My job was to convince publishers like Viacom to buy DRC's technology. An investor called me three hours into my first day of work: "Welcome to the team, Joey. We're thrilled to have you aboard. When do you think you'll have your first sale?" Sensing my amusement, he went on, "I wasn't joking, Joey. I'm very serious." The guy seemed a little stressed. As if his entire principal was at stake. The investors had just fired a bullet I was expected to outrun.

I immediately recruited Rebecca, now one of my best friends, who had left Questus in 2010 to take a senior-level position at a global agency, to be our vice president of strategic planning, and Cathy, whose resume included serving as chief marketing officer at a major headphone company, as our chief marketing officer. Over the next couple of months of focused effort, we crafted and presented proposals to a wide band of fascinated clients. By spring, the legal departments of two large commercial brands reviewed our proposed service contracts. But through the process of moving this company forward, I detected a number of contradictions between Tyler's assessment of our position and what I saw with my own eyes.

In March, I finally reviewed DRC's legal and financial filings, the company's disclosures related to assets, debts, revenue, and business expenses, tax returns, profit and loss statements, and promissory notes. DRC had not only failed to earn any consistent revenue in four years, but Tyler and his partner Mark had managed to burn through most of the $24 million in seed money with only a few promising beta studies with tiny populations to show for it. The heralded second phase of funding never materialized. Tyler had lied for the last two years, even at his son's birthday party. Lied to my face. My wife's face. In real life, DRC had no sustainable platform or infrastructure. Only a skeleton crew of developers and marketers. Inadequate research and case studies. No concrete evidence of scalability enabling huge short-term profits and an eventual IPO. On May 17th, 2014, DPC was closed by the board and investors. We were all terminated. I had plenty of time to think about my mistakes and feel guilty about their consequences. Like an aging boxer no longer able to avoid the most damaging punches, I contemplated retiring from the ring.

# Chapter 25

---

## Coach Joey
### (Present)

*Happiness is our natural state . . . the natural state of little children . . . Then why don't you experience it? Because you have to drop something. You've got to drop illusions . . . We need to put off the old man . . . When we start off in life, we look at reality with wonder . . . The wonder dies and is replaced by boredom, as we develop language and words and concepts.*

—Anthony de Mello

I own more clothing than Debbie, and prior to fatherhood, nobody caught me twice in the same outfit. Inconsistency was the rule. But last year, I acquired a piece of clothing I value more than any item in my tall, heavy closet: a dark-blue, lightweight polyester-and-rayon windbreaker, dabbed with snaps, priced in bulk, and manufactured for the San Francisco public school system, including Starr King Elementary. The windbreaker is sized for a larger man and imprinted with modest white lettering reading "Coach" on the left breast. I could not purchase it in a store. Like knighthood, I had to earn this one.

I never saw myself working with children in any capacity. Douchebags historically avoid helping professions such as K–12 education, firefighting, nursing, law enforcement, childcare, elder care, and youth athletics. Douchebags are not first responders. Or essential. Or heroes. We specialize in self-service, our performances better adapted for religious, political, and business stages where actions can hide behind the skirts of our words. We're the first one in the lifeboat. We are about adoration, attention, and acknowledgement. We absorb the applause. Not the hard work. About twenty years ago when I knew everything, as Paul blathered on about some life lesson he had discovered coaching "his kids," I interrupted with some derision, "Why do you think everything relates to gymnastics?" He looked at me like I was an idiot. Tried feeding me some hippie propaganda about shaping character through controlled adversity. If Paul and these children had learned so much, why was he making $10 an hour while I earned $50 an hour selling copy services? I felt kind of sorry for him.

When Kingston began attending Starr King Elementary School in 2017 (Kannon began the following year), our walks turned into forty-five-minute drives to and from Potrero Hill. Based on my constant presence and Kannon's zealous advocacy, Kingston and Kannon's stay-at-home dad was invited by the teachers to act as Joey Chaperone. Docent Joey. I helped out with trips to museums. Chinatown. Parks. Playgrounds. School events and celebrations. I had a blast. I never had so much fun earning so little money. San Francisco's public school recreation program further offered ongoing six-week soccer, basketball, and baseball seasons throughout the school year that allowed every student to participate, which resulted in a desperate need for parent-volunteer coaches. The job description said it all, parent being the prerequisite rank, the true stakeholders, those with true love for the game. No proxies. No pinch hitters. No promissory notes. The boys and I signed up for every sport.

I was not an academic or an artist when I was young. But I was good at sports. Scores of them. My active participation in athletic contests, schoolyard and sanctioned, provided me abundant physical, social, and economic fitness advantages throughout my life. Joey Captain. Top Draft Joey. Joey Starter. I always played. No game without me. Paul typed up a list once—it included everything from archery to dirt bikes to trampoline, stopping at forty-five activities that met the standard of performing competently in front of people. Of playing at a level where others wanted you on the team. Certainly, my boys and their classmates would be awed by SportsCenter Joey's laser-brilliant pointers and epic sports stories. A modern-day Aesop in Adidas sportswear and designer aviator sunglasses. Joey Buck. Air Joey. How lucky were these children?

I learned my first day as a soccer coach that little boys were crazy. Lego brains with some assembly required. Hilarious, adorable, and worth the effort, but ruled by fire's immediacy and primal instinct. Dangerous. Loud. Explosive. Desperate for contact and consequences. Hard of hearing. Couldn't tie their shoes. They ran into each other. Threw things at each other's eyes. Wrestled on dirty floors. Offered insensitive observations at inopportune moments. Kicked and broke stuff. I was lucky if I held their attention for twenty seconds before the chatter, giggling, and goosing began to interfere with my precise instructional points related to movement and spacing. They were not interested in my stories. My words and phrases had to be few and proud like the Marines.

Luckily, I had a lot of help. All of the team parents contributed, from contacting to snacking. Coaching colleagues Tom and Troy, like me, were raised in the Midwest amidst gophers, badgers, and wolverines, where sports were revered as rites of passage portending manly survival, fertility, and heroic legacies, and lesser men got their lesser butts kicked for not fighting hard enough. Coaching involved a lot of talking. Proud talk. Discipline talk. Technical talk. Inspirational talk. Our language formed a variety of shapes and sounds to achieve a variety of purposes: teacher, choreographer, referee, nurse, psychologist, timekeeper, mediator, and security guard to a dozen or so kinetic children. Researchers who observed and categorized legendary Coach John Wooden's acts of communication during a UCLA basketball practice session found that he spent 75 percent of them giving specific instruction, 12 percent demanding hustle, 7 percent passing along praise, and 6 percent scolding poor performance.

My coaching sentences needed nametags. Command of each child's carefully chosen name was as close to a magical protective spell as nature could cast for imparting knowledge, guidance, and feedback. Schools take roll every hour for a reason. "Kingston, pay attention!" "Jack, today you were the MVP!" A teacher's silence was not golden. Silence was derelict and lazy. Truth must be told, not implied. "Marco, you did a great job of challenging Stuart Hall's forwards at midfield." "I'm proud of you, Kannon." While nonverbal cues and expressions serve important roles in all communication, teaching, like music, must be heard to move us. "Jimmy, drop back and cut off the passing lane." "Jaden, keep your hands to yourself!" Reasonable minds differ on the appropriate level of volume, from easy listening to rage metal. Speaking for my coaching colleagues, we preferred rock and roll with the bass cranked up. We got carried away sometimes and have the yellow cards to prove it. We cared like fans.

While each athlete was a separate spirit, patterns emerged as the kids acclimated to the demands of the sport. Part of my job was to identify and integrate these patterns into precise points of instruction. I spent a lot of time watching and listening. Jack and Justin were pretty good listeners. Marco and Jaden were brawlers. Kingston and Justin were two of the league's scoring leaders. Alex and Kannon were power forwards. Michael and Max were speedsters. Jimmy and Michael muscled the middle and guarded the goal. Kingston and Marco covered the entire field. Luke and Theo liked to play goalie. I learned which boys were distracted by shiny objects, and which of them was likely to trip over untied laces, draw a penalty out of anger, get caught out of position, make a penalty shot, sit back on his heels, get caught offside, pass to an opposing player, or inspire the team. Not so difficult to sort out. Once I paid attention.

Our opponent at the last game was a team we tied 2-2 earlier in our undefeated season. Winner took all. I felt anxious and crabby for no good reason. The boys played magnificently, prevailing 6-1. We had to bench Kingston for scoring five goals in the first half. I don't hate to brag. Shared joy spilled all over the place. More than anyone of us could contain. Players and families hooted and hollered. Replayed highlights on the drives home. Dreamed bigger dreams that night. Stored emergency flashlight memories of a chilly championship afternoon for future night hikes. All this, despite my minor supporting role. How cool was that? In exchange for good faith, I earned spectacular returns. It took me over forty years to recognize that my self-worth could not skyrocket until I started investing in others. The douchebag believes he can obtain nourishment by consuming himself. Most of us are slow learners.

I'm curious again. Fascinated with my family. Proud. Reliant. Infused. Enthused. Often bewildered, rarely certain, and stoked to be in love with living. If you get over to yellow-bricked Russian Hill on a sunny afternoon, you might spot a rare recovering douchebag, the smiling man in the yellow hat who holds his children's hands and looks both ways before he crosses the street.

***

## Epilogue

---

## Joey Vulnerability

Kingston and Kannon are fascinated by Stan Lee's fictional American superhero, Iron Man, especially the films released in 2008, 2010, and 2013 starring Robert Downey, Jr. Fast-paced plots incorporate cool sci-fi technology, black-hearted villainy, witty dialogue, and digitized seat-shaking thermodynamic collisions. A stack of vintage Iron Man comics evicted Dr. Seuss from his high-rise bookshelf space in their bedroom. Deeply versed in Marvel Comics nerd-lore, Uncle Paul leads discussions of Iron Man's biography and development dating back to the character's first appearance in 1963. Years later, I still enjoy the bi-monthly screenings.

Debbie tolerates the choreographed violence because the Iron Man saga has palpably stoked Kingston and Kannon's respect and excitement for chemistry, physics, technology, electrical engineering, and even psychology. A few months ago, both boys memorized the periodic table of elements, all 118. One Saturday morning, I found them studying elements under a microscope. They want circuit board kits, Bunsen burners, Erlenmeyer flasks, and alkali metals. I field continuous questions about everything I never learned in school. Is his suit really made of iron? What is palladium and how does it power the arc reactor? Why did Iron Man freeze when he flew too high? How fast was he falling? They wonder about the complex man sealed within his magical armor, genius inventor billionaire industrialist Tony Stark. Is Tony smart? Does he like himself too much? How does he know so much about machines? What does MIT stand for? What is wrong with Tony?

Iron Man 3 contains several scenes depicting Tony Stark's stress-induced, recurring, and immobilizing panic attacks. My hometown Mayo Clinic characterizes anxiety as toxic in high doses, manifesting as repeated episodes of sudden, intense, excessive, and persistent worry, fear, terror, and dread that can escalate and peak within minutes. Chronic, difficult to control, and disproportionate to actual danger, the physiological and psychological effects of anxiety can originate during childhood and continue into adulthood, reaching the level of a disorder when its symptoms objectively interfere with the sufferer's daily activities. Some survivors require medication and psychotherapy.

I was touched by Robert Downey, Jr.'s raw portrayal of Stark's untreated anxiety disorder: the vise-pressured accelerating heart rate, reverberating paranoia, constricted blood vessels and bouncing vision, crashing and debilitating racetrack thoughts. Observing Tony Stark's emotional fragility, no longer hidden behind the invincibility of his vaunted armor, felt tragic and authentic. Familiar and validating. Within these frames, I watched Downey, Jr. act out my pain. He named it. Portrayed the courage to accept it. If most of our battles are fought within ourselves, does it really matter whether acts of heroism are inspired by reality or fiction? None of this was lost on our boys.

This book has caused me to recall, with more honesty, my continuing struggle with anxiety, including my first panic attacks in 1981 catalyzed by the domestic violence dynamics of Dad's dark household. The frequent fights when I doused fear with aggression. The sloshing mental-anguish midnights that wore me out. Decades of self-aggrandizing egocentric overreach and open-throttled near-suicide motorcycle rides. Bad boyfriend behavior and cutthroat capitalism. My soul shielded by my weaponized armor of ego. The Iron Douche-bag.

There will be no quick fixes. I have a lot to learn. From books, from other people, and from long walks inside my own consciousness. Nobody is invulnerable and nobody is unafraid. I am in good company. Ready. At attention. I continue to plumb and dislodge memories of deep-pressured moments and heart-bursting joys, failures and triumphs and the life in between. I now recognize the many life lessons that make me look upward. Reminding me of somebody I used to know.